Sedation in De

Sedation in Dentistry

N.M. Girdler PhD BDS BSc FDSRCS FFDRCS

and

C.M. Hill MDSc FDSRCS LDSRCS BDS MSc

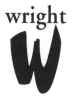

wright

EDINBURGH LONDON NEW YORK OXFORD PHILADELPHIA ST LOUIS SYDNEY TORONTO 1998

Wright
An imprint of Elsevier Science Limited

First published 1998
Reprinted 2000, 2002, 2003

British Library Cataloguing in Publication Data
A catalogue record for this book is available from the British Library

Library of Congress Cataloging in Publication Data
A catalog record for this book is available from the Library of Congress

ISBN 0 7236 1052 5

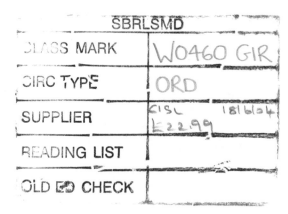
Printed and bound by MPG Books Ltd, Bodmin, Cornwall

Contents

Foreword

As yet, the decline in general anaesthesia, despite the recommendations of the 1990 'Report of the Working Party on General Anaesthesia, Sedation and Resuscitation in Dentistry', has failed to be realized, and 'Dental Phobia' still exists. In addition, the expected increase in simple sedation using intravenous midazolam has also only been realized to a small extent in general dental practice, although more so in hospital practice. Perhaps this pattern reflects the long lag period between the introduction of good clinical instruction in using inhalation or intravenous sedation in dental teaching hospitals and the application of this excellent method of dealing with frightened dental patients in dental practice.

This text is a model instruction manual for all who wish to improve their knowledge of pharmacology, clinical applications and methods of use of all forms of sedation. It covers the whole subject in a seamless fashion, from basic science to the application of sedation in everyday practice, whether in dental hospital departments or general or specialist practice. It should also be read and welcomed by trainee anaesthetists and gastroenterologists who are regularly using anaesthesia and sedation in their daily practice. Both authors have considerable experience of sedation, local anaesthesia, resuscitation and the rare but significant complications of sedation. They do not neglect either end of the spectrum of special knowledge which begins with relevant physiology and pharmacology, taking the reader rapidly and painlessly through the practical techniques to the worst complication any practitioner can have—medical negligence litigation.

Not all textbooks are concise, easy to read and contain, especially in the clinical practice section, authoritative information for practitioners at all levels of seniority. This book is interesting to read, easy to understand and adequately illustrated. It should be welcomed by all who wish to treat dental phobic patients and to assist them in overcoming their fear of dental and minor oral surgical treatment under local analgesia.

The authors should be congratulated on this concise, practical manual which carries the stamp of quality and authority. They have succeeded in updating the 'Poswillo' report in the light of the very considerable changes, especially in resuscitation, drugs and procedures which have occurred world-wide since 1990.

Professor David Poswillo CBE

Preface

Over the past decade, conscious sedation has become a topical subject in the field of dental 'anaesthesia'. The publication of the Department of Health Working Party Report—colloquially referred to as the Poswillo Report—in 1990 stimulated many dental surgeons to look away from general anaesthesia as a means of treating anxious patients towards alternative methods of anxiety control.

Building on a sound understanding of behavioural management, we have attempted to produce a concise account of sedation as it relates to the practice of dentistry. Wherever possible, we have tried to start with fairly basic foundations in order to build a sound understanding of the principles and practice of administering safe sedation. The wider application of sedation in premedication is also considered so that dentists may be aware of the scope of modern-day practice in a hospital environment as well as in the dental surgery.

An increasing awareness amongst patients and the advent of modern sedation methods has meant that there is a wealth of material which could be included in a book of this nature. Above all, we hope that this book will be a readable account which will satisfy the demands of undergraduates and qualified dentists for training in sedation techniques. It should provide the theoretical basis from which practical skills can be learnt.

Acknowledgements

We would like to acknowledge the kind and long-suffering support of our wives and families during the preparation of this book. To our colleagues who have given constructive criticism and endless encouragement, our thanks are also due.

The audiovisual departments at the University of Newcastle-upon-Tyne and the University Dental Hospital NHS Trust in Cardiff have given us much assistance in the preparation of many of the photographs and illustrations and we are very grateful for their help. Figures 6.1, 6.2, 6.4, 6.6–6.11, 6.13, 6.14, 6.16, 6.18, 8.1, 8.2, 8.4–8.8 and 8.11–8.20 are reproduced with kind permission of the University of Newcastle-upon-Tyne who retain copyright ownership. Figure 6.3 has been revised and reproduced with kind permission of the Royal College of Surgeons of England. Figure 8.10 was provided by and used with the kind permission of Laerdal UK.

Finally, our thanks are due to all our students—past and present—whose stimulation and interest has been the driving force to enable us to complete this project. Thank you all.

Spectrum of patient management

Introduction

The purpose of this chapter is to present a framework for the management of dental patients and to give an understanding of the rationale behind the methods used in treating anxious patients. In order to achieve this, it is necessary to understand why people behave in the way they do in coping well with stressful situations, whilst others seem to be able to tolerate very little. It is also useful to know how behaviour can be modified in a way that is beneficial for both the patient and the dentist. This can often be achieved without resorting to the use of drugs so as to allow long-term solutions to acute problems of behavioural management. Where this is possible it is nearly always preferable to methods of sedation which rely on the use of drugs since any drug, virtually by definition, will have some undesirable side effects. In addition there is good evidence that patients actually adapt to the use of sedation and become dependent on it despite this being contrary to one of the first principles of sedation, i.e. to rehabilitate anxious patients so that they can contemplate conventional treatment. The first chapter of this book therefore concentrates on patient management and behavioural under-standing.

Perception and sensation

Contrary to many people's understanding perception and sensation are not the same entity. Historically, five principal senses were described which convey information to the brain. These are touch, taste, smell, sight and hearing; the sensation of pain is undoubtedly a sixth sensation and should now be added to the list.

Sensation may be defined as the ability of the brain to receive a particular experience resulting from the stimulation of one of the sensory organs. The main part of the mechanism, however, is the process by which the brain detects and interprets information from its sensory receptors. Sensory information is not simply received passively; the brain intuitively analyses and interprets sensory information and formulates a response based on such an interpretation. The responses are to a large extent predictable and repeatable and this begins to define what is meant by behaviour. The awareness of sensation is termed 'perception' which can be defined as the process by which sensory information is analysed and made meaningful. This is far less constant and predictable than a simple response to a single sensory stimulus and adds another dimension to the concept of behaviour.

The neurological processes that determine sensation, perception and response are highly complicated and vary from a simple reflex action to a complex, rationalized, cortical response. Why perception varies so considerably between individuals is the subject of a good number of psychological theories. The simplest of these is the bottom-up theories of which there are several models, which argue that perception is simply a result of sensory stimulation. Conversely, top-down theories emphasize the fundamental importance of prior knowledge and other cognitive factors in perceptive response. Whichever theory is adopted, however, there is general agreement that perception plays a large part in the establishment of personality and behaviour which are themselves both inter-related.

Behaviour

Behaviour may be defined as functioning in a specified, predictable or normal way. In psychological terms behaviour is a response or series of responses of a person to a given stimulus. Behavioural theory, however, generally tends to refer to the behaviour of an individual in terms of comparison with a majority. The borderline between what is normal (or acceptable) and abnormal (or unacceptable) behaviour is blurred by a host of factors including time, culture, conditioning and other considerations.

Significant deviation from normal behaviour has been classified in different ways, the most commonly accepted method being that of Kraepelin (1913) (Table 1.1). Fundamentally, this divides mental disorder into neurotic and psychotic abnormality of which there are many different variants. A simple way of identifying the two principal types is to understand the neurotic person as one who calculates $2 + 2 = 4$ and is extremely concerned about the result. A psychotic person, for example, will calculate $2 + 2 = 5$, but will have no concern about this whatsoever.

Neurosis therefore tends to lead towards such conditions as phobias and obsessive compulsions, whereas psychosis may lead to loss of reality, schizophrenia and delusory behaviour. Concerns about reality are neurotic whilst those relating to unreality or delusion are psychotic.

There is one other aspect of behaviour that needs to be considered, however, and that is to understand why people actually respond the way they do. In 1980, Ajzen and Fishbein developed what they termed the theory of reasoned action. This is based on an understanding that healthy people will behave in a rational and sensible way once they have taken into account the information available to them and the implication of their actions (or lack of action).

Ajzen and Fishbein would claim that how a person intends to act is more informative than their apparent or expressed attitudes when it comes to predicting how they will respond. They would argue that intentions are a combination of two factors. First, a person's attitude towards a behaviour

Table 1.1 Kraepelin's 'medical model' of abnormal behaviour

Classification	Symptom
Neuroses	Disorders which involve excessive anxiety in 'normal' situations. Anxiety is usually contained by the person avoiding its source, which can lead to odd behaviour at times. Neuroses may develop into phobias, an obsessive compulsion or even a case of multiple personality. (Multiple personality is often called 'schizophrenia' in popular speech, but is actually quite different from the clinical disorder known as schizophrenia)
Personality disorders	This is a category of mental disorder where thinking processes are socially unusual or deviant. They include paranoia, obsessive personality, schizoid personality and psychopathy. Psychopaths are not necessarily criminals or under psychiatric care. They are also found in careers which value such attributes, such as entertainment, politics or big business, and can be extremely likeable people
Organic psychoses	These disorders are the result of identifiable physical causes, such as brain tumours, injuries to the nervous system or degenerative neural disease like Huntington's chorea or infective diseases such as tertiary syphilis. Organic psychoses are relatively rare after cerebrovascular accidents
Functional psychoses	Functional psychoses are those in which the person is clearly disturbed and not in touch with reality but where there is no apparent organic cause. Kraepelin described two general types of functional psychosis: schizophrenia and manic-depressive psychosis
Mental retardation	This is not actually a mental illness, but it was classified by Kraepelin as a mental disorder. Mentally retarded patients were characterized in this system by an extreme slowness to respond to stimuli, a general lack of interest or curiosity and low IQ scores

pattern rather than the stimulus itself and second, their perception of social or cultural pressure to respond or not respond in a certain fashion. This they termed 'subjective normality' and it goes some way towards explaining why behavioural management in children and adolescents is such a different problem from the behavioural management of adults. Put another way, the intent of adults would most commonly be to want to behave in a rational and sensible manner, whereas the same intent would not always be present in children and adolescents. It therefore follows that the management of what appears to be similar but abnormal behaviour in the different groups needs to be tackled from a different viewpoint. This illustrates the complexity of the problem when it comes to teaching or learning techniques of behavioural management.

In conclusion, it can be seen that behaviour is a complex issue governed by a multitude of factors, some of which are illustrated in Figure 1.1. Equally, the management of behaviour is a difficult and extensive subject and features largely in several common textbooks of psychology. However, the successful treatment of any patient depends on a dentist's ability to manage his or her behaviour satisfactorily and some of the techniques of behavioural management are discussed below.

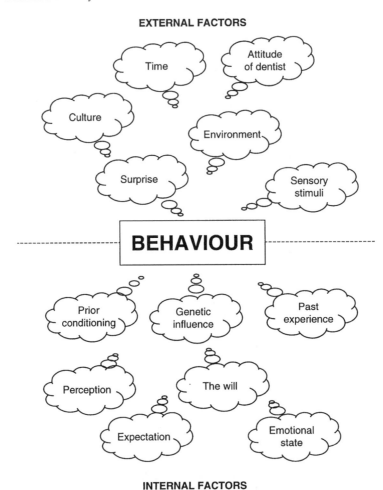

Figure 1.1 Some of the factors influencing behaviour.

Behavioural management

Simple methods

There is an element of fear in all unknown situations in the majority of normal individuals. Probably the most important aspect of behavioural management is to ensure that the provoking stimulus is minimized as far as possible. Much of this is common sense and includes paying attention to such factors as room decoration, the way staff are dressed, the playing of gentle music in the background, etc.

In addition, positive distraction can be applied with the use of ceiling television and dedicated Walkman headphones for example. Although the five sensations of sight, sound, hearing, touch and smell can all be offensive to patients in the dental surgery, it is undoubtedly the fear of pain which is the most commonly quoted factor which inhibits individuals seeking treatment or which underlies the apparently irrational behaviour of many anxious patients.

In such patients, simple behavioural management consists of informing verbally and demonstrating practically before actually performing a procedure. This has commonly been interpreted as a 'tell, show, do' sequence and there is good evidence that it is effective in many people. It does, however, depend on patients being able to adopt a rational approach to unknown situations. It is unlikely to be very effective in phobic patients or those demonstrating other types of neurotic behaviour.

Another simple method of behavioural management, and one which is particularly suitable for use in children, is sometimes referred to as 'permissible deception'. An example of this would be the introduction of an infiltration local anaesthetic into an upper premolar region without a patient being told they were having an injection and without them observing the needle. Providing adequate topical anaesthesia has first been obtained and the needle is not seen by the patient, abnormal behavioural responses are rarely seen in such situations. In such techniques, it is important not to tell lies but to be 'economical with the truth' using such terms as squirting some numbing water, washing the gums or making the teeth go to sleep. Successful application of these simple techniques is highly dependent on the confidence of the person applying them. The success of the administration can then be used as a building block on which further steps can be built.

Behavioural response is also heightened by stress and simple relaxation techniques can be applied to enable tense patients to relax. This may be achieved actively (Figure 1.2) or passively by using soft background music for example.

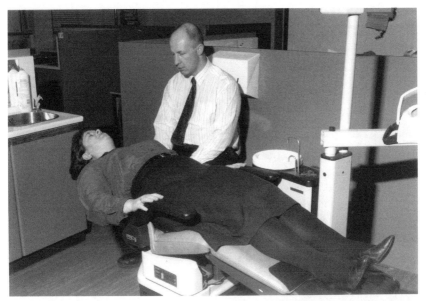

Figure 1.2 A patient relaxing whilst concentrating on regular breathing whilst counting backwards from 1000 in steps of seven. This method can be adapted to from the basis of a simple means of hypnotic induction.

It has also been shown that patients perceive the degree of stress being experienced by the dentist and respond accordingly developing heightened responses to any stimuli. It is therefore essential that dentists review their own responses in difficult or stressful situations and take every action possible to moderate them accordingly.

Finally, it is possible to use biofeedback techniques to teach relaxation. Using sound or visual equipment, biofeedback involves teaching people a degree of control over their autonomic responses. Typically when measuring pulse rate, blood pressure or muscular activity a biofeedback machine (Figure 1.3) will produce a higher or louder tone when activity increases. Patients then concentrate on lowering the activity level by applying positive relaxation. Like many of these relaxation techniques it is very effective in some people and others seem to find it impossible to control their responses.

Conditioning techniques

There are two classic conditioning techniques used in the treatment of phobic patients of which the first (systematic desensitization) is the most common and potentially most effective. This technique involves gradually acclimatizing patients to very minor stimuli and teaching them to relax whilst they are being applied. Once relaxation is achieved the stimulus can be gradually increased usually over a considerable period of time until even the most feared situation is manageable.

Many dentists intuitively use this approach in treating extremely anxious patients, first of all introducing a mirror and then a probe followed by the use of hand-scalers, tooth-brushing with the dental engine, maxillary infiltration, small

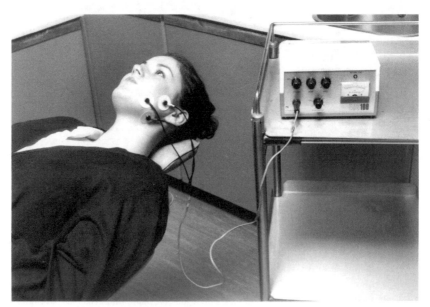

Figure 1.3 A patient using a biofeedback machine to aid relaxation. The effect is partly due to genuine relaxation and partly to the distracting noise of the machine bleeping.

restoration, inferior dental block, etc. In many cases it is possible to teach a new set of learnt behaviours, replacing the previously maladapted ones.

A second and more extreme form of conditioning, and one which is not commonly used in the profession, is known as 'implosion therapy'. In such cases a prolonged and increasing exposure to the fear stimulus is initiated in order to try and produce habituation. The principle behind these techniques is that initial panic is gradually replaced by a progressive reduction in fear, thus disassociating the relationship between the fear and the stimulus itself.

Various other techniques have been used in all sorts of differing situations. A common approach in the late twentieth century has been the establishment of self-help support groups and Crawford et al. (1997) reported on the qualitative assessment of the effectiveness of such a group. Their key messages were that members who attended the group felt (at least initially) that their anxiety was abnormal and isolated them from 'normal' members of society. In addition, attendance at the group dissipated anxiety and promoted feelings of empathy and confidence. The support was also demonstrably effective in enabling patients to actually complete their treatment but the cost was in the dependence the group members developed in the dentist group leader.

Finally, mention should be made of the various counselling techniques which are available today. Initially inspired by the work of Sigmund Freud, they are largely a product of the late twentieth century. These techniques are often subjective and largely untested other than being extrapolated from a particular theory of psychology. The most commonly employed therapy techniques are Cognitive, Rogerian, Gestalt, Personal Construct, Rational Emotive, Transactional Analysis and Family Therapy but there are many more—each with its proponents and opponents. Counselling therapy can be effective but it is not always predictable and it can be very time consuming.

Hypnosis

The use of hypnosis in dentistry has been slowly increasing as more scientific research and effective post-graduate training have shown the potential benefits of this technique. This growth has not occurred easily as hypnosis has always been a somewhat controversial subject! In the middle ages it was condemned by the church and by conventional practitioners of medicine and its use in some circumstances is still highly questionable. Therapeutic hypnosis has not been helped by the emergence of stage hypnotists who use and manipulate susceptible people by inducing deep hypnotic trances and making them 'perform' in ways which their inhibitory reactions would normally prevent.

None-the-less there are occasions when hypnosis can be used in anxious patients to considerable benefit. This may take the simple form of a light hypnotic trance which creates an illusion of relaxation and remoteness (rather like the feeling of a Sunday afternoon nap!) to the use of more complicated phenomena, such as hypno-analgesia, where the effects of a local anaesthetic can be induced through suggestion alone.

Hypnosis is generally believed to be one of the 'altered states'—a situation of 'altered' consciousness rather than alertness or unconsciousness. Sleep is the best known and most common of the altered states and, in terms of EEG activity, there are some similarities, as well as considerable differences, between sleep and hypnosis. It should be noted that there are some theorists who do not believe that hypnosis is a 'state' but that it is a social phenomenon, explicable in terms of socio-psychological responses.

It has been suggested that in a hypnotic state patients never act against their own consciences and always co-operate voluntarily with their hypnotist. This theory must be open to question after the conviction of a 'therapeutic hypnotist' on charges of rape, committed whilst he had deeply hypnotized a patient who succeeded in proving in a court of law that she had acted against her own will.

Over the years there have been various theories of hypnosis, none of which entirely satisfies all the known criteria of the hypnotic state. However, in essence hypnotic phenomena can be divided into five groups:

1. *Ability enhancement*—an ability to undertake tasks not previously thought possible.
2. *Memory variation*—an ability to retain, recall or reject information.
3. *Pain control*—an ability to relieve pain in a clinical environment.
4. *Age regression*—an ability to revert to an earlier part of a person's life.
5. *A hidden observer*—a perception that one half of the mind is observing what the other half is doing during the hypnotized state.

Induction of the hypnotic state can be performed verbally (or by use of non-spoken sound), visually or by the patients themselves. The details of possible techniques are to be found in several books on hypnosis but they all rely on inducing a trance-like state by unreasoned action. Thus a person may be asked to concentrate on an oblique corner, listen to certain music, imagine a journey or follow a pattern of relaxation. There are also methods of inducing ultra-rapid trances which are very effective in susceptible subjects. Once the hypnotic state is induced it can be deepened in a variety of ways depending on the application required.

In dentistry the purpose of hypnosis is to facilitate treatment rather than as a therapeutic technique. It may also be used for that purpose but its principal uses are listed by Chaves (1997) who summarizes ten possible uses of hypnosis in dentistry—all of which are treatment orientated.

A detailed treatise on the subject of hypnosis is outside the scope of this book but it is a technique which has not been exploited fully by the profession and one which deserves further consideration.

Sedation

Despite all the techniques of behavioural management and alternative methods it is still the case that there remains a large number of people who, despite all reasonable attempts to manage their behaviour without the use of drugs, feel unable to undertake dental treatment without some form of drug therapy. Up to 45% of adults in the UK claim that fear is their reason for non-attendance at the dentist (Todd and Lader, 1991). Of this number, it is estimated that one-third are severely anxious (phobic) and two-thirds are moderately anxious. In the course of this book the various means by which sedation can be delivered will be considered but it should be mentioned that even the administration of a placebo has been found to be effective in up to 30% of patients. It is, therefore, possible to adopt a stepped approach to patient management—first attempting simple behavioural management techniques and subsequently moving along the scale to

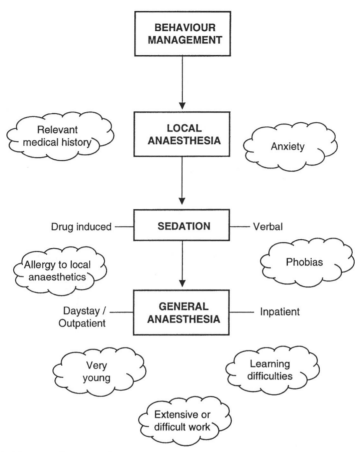

Figure 1.4 A progressive approach to patient management and the factors which influence decision making.

sedation or even general anaesthesia in a few cases. This is represented in Figure 1.4 with suggestions as to the sort of factors which influence decision making. It is unlikely that a definitive algorithm of treatment choice can be produced but it is certainly helpful to think along the lines of progressing along a route rather than adopting a two-way decision process which often occurs. There is good evidence that this will be beneficial in the long term since patients who have general anaesthesia or profound sedation from the outset are less likely to attend recall appointments and have a higher incidence of subsequent dental disease. Those who adopt a progressive approach to sedation, with a view to using it as a treatment modality which can gradually be reduced, are more likely to be successful in their treatment of anxious patients. Sedation should therefore be considered in severely anxious (phobic) patients, moderately anxious patients, those undergoing difficult or prolonged procedures, anxious child patients, those with certain physical or mental handicap and those who may otherwise require a general anaesthetic.

Local anaesthesia

This is not a book on the subject of local anaesthesia but the whole subject of pain control and behavioural management is, as was mentioned earlier, very closely linked. Whilst the fear of pain remains the prime reason for people failing to attend the dentist the linkage is likely to remain. The experience of pain evokes an emotional response and this frequently appears to be disproportionate to the applied stimulus. This lack of proportion is sometimes seen in a diminished form (e.g. a person allowing a dental extraction to be completed without any local anaesthetic being administered) but more commonly it is exaggerated, for example with loud screaming or tears flooding down the cheeks after an apparently minor painful stimulus.

It is, therefore, important to emphasize the need for effective local anaesthesia since it is the cornerstone of pain-free dental treatment in the vast majority of individuals who seek and obtain dental treatment.

Failure to achieve analgesia is rarely due to psychosomatic intention on the part of the patient and failures are usually due to anatomical, pharmacological or pathological reasons. At the one end of the spectrum such reasons may simply be due to depositing the local anaesthetic in the wrong place (common with failed inferior dental blocks) whilst at the other, it may be due to the complex histochemical reactions that occur when infection is present.

Whatever the cause, local anaesthesia is used to supplement sedation in the majority of cases and an efficient and effective technique in local anaesthesia is essential. It is especially salutary to remember that no amount of sedation will compensate for inadequate analgesia and several serious adverse events have been documented when clinicians have failed to realize this fact. The answer to inadequate local anaesthesia is better local anaesthesia—**not** more sedation!

General anaesthesia

Finally, within the spectrum of patient management, the subject of general anaesthesia needs to be briefly discussed. Modern sedation has undoubtedly reduced the number of those patients who require a general anaesthetic to tolerate dental treatment but there remains a significant number who seem unable to tolerate the idea of treatment of any sort unless they are rendered totally unconscious. For this group of people no amount of talking or even persuasion will make any difference; unless they are 'knocked out' they will not have any treatment even regardless of the degree of pain they are suffering. Whilst this may appear totally irrational (and is!) it is no less real and it must be accepted that for those people, a caring profession must provide anaesthetic services at least for the relief of pain and other emergency dental situations. This was the basis of the Department of Health Report in 1990, more commonly referred to as the Poswillo Report. Where general anaesthetic services are provided, they must be to the same high standard as found in district and teaching hospitals; there can be no room for any compromise on grounds of safety. Poswillo also recommended that sedation should be used in preference to general anaesthesia whenever possible, advice which appears to have had only limited acceptance.

Since the Department of Health Report, the General Dental Council have twice amended their regulations regarding sedation and anaesthesia and the current advice is reproduced in Figure 1.5. In addition, the Royal College of Surgeons of

4.8 RISKS OF GENERAL ANAESTHESIA

General Anaesthesia is a procedure which is never without risk. In assessing the needs of the individual patient due regard should be given to all aspects of behavioural management and anxiety control before deciding to proceed with general anaesthesia.

A DENTIST WHO CARRIES OUT TREATMENT UNDER GENERAL ANAESTHESIA OR SEDATION WITHOUT ENSURING THAT THE CONDITIONS SET OUT BELOW ARE MET IS LIABLE TO A CHARGE OF SERIOUS PROFESSIONAL MISCONDUCT.

4.9 FULL MEDICAL HISTORY AND CONSENT

Prior to the administration of general anaesthesia or sedation, a full medical history of the patient must be taken and consent obtained. Patients must be given in advance clear and comprehensive pre- and post-operative instructions in writing. Careful contemporaneous records of treatment and the procedure undertaken must also be kept.

4.12 ASSISTANCE DURING CONSCIOUS SEDATION

Where conscious sedation techniques are employed a suitable experienced denstist may assume the responsibility of sedating the patient as well as operating, providing that the relevant post-graduate training has been undertaken. As a minimum requirement a second appropriately trained person must be present throughout who is capable of monitoring the clinical condition of the patient and of assisting the dentist in the event of an emergency.

4.13 DEFINITION OF SEDATION

Conscious sedation may be defined as:

'A technique in which the use of a drug or drugs produces a state of depression of the central nervous system enabling treatment to be carried out, but during which communication can be maintained and the modification of the patient's state of mind is such that the patient will respond to command throughout the period of sedation. Techniques used should carry a margin of safety wide enough to render unintended loss of consciousness unlikely.'

4.14 DRUG USE, MONITORING AND RESUSCITATION

The technique chosen should be the most appropriate to enable successful treatment to be given and in the case of intravenous sedation will normally be by the use of a single drug. Contemporary standards of monitoring should be adopted during conscious sedation and where more than one sedative drug is utilised the provision of advanced life support must be immediately available. The current guidelines issued by the Resuscitation Council (UK) are also appropriate in this connection.

4.15 INTRAVENOUS SEDATION AND CHILDREN

The effect of intravenous sedation is unpredictable in children. The therapeutic margin between sedation and anaesthesia may be very narrow and there is always the possibility of a paradoxical reaction. In view of this, intravenous sedation in children should be administered only in very special circumstances.

4.16 RECOVERY AND DISCHARGE

Patients who are recovering from general anaesthesia or sedation should be appropriately protected and monitored in adequate recovery facilities. When . . . the patient is sufficiently recovered to leave the premises they should be accompanied by a responsible adult. The only situation in which a dentist may exercise discretion as to whether an adult patient may be discharged unaccompanied is when nitrous oxide/oxygen sedation alone has been used. All patients must be specifically assessed for discharge.

4.17 EQUIPMENT, FACILITIES AND TRAINING

Neither general anaesthesia nor sedation should be employed unless proper equipment for their administration is used and adequate recovery facilities, including appropriate drugs for resuscitation of the patient are readily available with both the dentist and staff trained in the . . . techniques.

4.18 COLLAPSE

Since the administration of general anaesthesia or sedation may increase the risk of collapse, a dentist should ensure that all members of the dental team are properly trained and prepared to deal with an emergency. Training should include frequent practice of resuscitation routines in a simulated emergency.

Figure 1.5 Extracts from the current General Dental Council regulations (1997) (*reproduced by kind permission*).

England established a joint working party which produced a report (1993) which more specifically addressed the practice of sedation by non-anaesthetists.

The whole question of sedation and anaesthesia is still high on the political agenda and it is inevitable that further developments will occur over the next few years. These are likely to result in the need for more intensive post-graduate training for those wishing to carry out sedation in general practice. It is also likely that only medically-trained anaesthetists will be allowed to administer general anaesthetics, possibly in licensed or regulated premises.

The history of sedation

It is difficult to pinpoint the beginnings of sedation from a historical point of view. The uses of alcohol as a narcoleptic is mentioned in the old testament of the Bible and there is evidence that opiates were used in the centuries before Christ in the eastern world. Modern sedation, however, has evolved over the last hundred years. In the preceding century the practice of anaesthesia itself had been established and popularized. This followed the discovery of nitrous oxide by Joseph Priestley in 1776 who himself described the effects produced as 'an highly pleasurable thrilling'.

Some twenty years later Humphry Davy observed the analgesic properties of nitrous oxide and suggested that it would be suitable for use in surgical procedures. His proposal was largely ignored until Horace Wells, a dental surgeon of Connecticut, USA, used nitrous oxide to extract a tooth. Whether the effect he originally obtained was one of anaesthesia or relative analgesia will possibly never be known for certain. Since he employed the technique on himself prior to using it on his patients, it could be assumed that the effect was one of sedation rather than anaesthesia.

Historically, a number of intravenous drugs have also been used for sedation. Many of the original 'sedation' agents were really general anaesthetic drugs used in smaller doses to try and produce a state of sedation. The drugs included cocktails such as phenobarbitone, pethidine and scopolamine (the Jorgensen technique—named after Danish Professor Nils Jorgensen). Another technique was popularized by the late Drummond-Jackson and involved giving (allegedly) sub-anaesthetic, multiple doses of the barbiturate methohexitone to induce 'twilight sleep'. Thiopentone, a similar but slightly more potent barbiturate anaesthetic, has also been used in this regard.

Needless to say, the margin between sedation and anaesthesia was so close that mishaps were inevitable and the practice of intermittent methohexitone was largely discontinued in the early 1970s after one or two fatal episodes. The problem remained that the distinction between sedation and general anaesthesia with all these agents was extremely narrow and they therefore carried a very fine margin of safety. Accidental anaesthesia with all its attendant dangers was not uncommon.

The fact that sedation practice has largely superseded anaesthetic practice in the UK was due in no small part to the synthesis of a class of drugs now widely known as the benzodiazepines. The first of these, chlordiazepoxide, was synthesized in 1956 but it was the introduction of diazepam—Valium® (see Appendix 1 for list of trade names and UK suppliers)—in both oral and parenteral forms which really heralded the arrival of safe conscious sedation.

Continued development of sedation techniques has progressed steadily over the past 30 years. Synthesis of the various benzodiazepines has been accompanied with excellent research into their mode of action and this is discussed later in Chapter 4. During this period also there have been several attempts to regulate the growth of sedation and to ensure its safe practice.

In 1978, the first national report on sedation in the UK was produced under the chairmanship of Dr John Wylie. Its most famous achievement was to formulate a definition for conscious sedation which was to become the bedrock of the future development. Conscious sedation was defined as: 'A technique in which the use of a drug or drugs produces a state of depression of the central nervous system enabling treatment to be carried out, but during which verbal contact is maintained with the patient at all times. The margin of safety of the drugs must be wide enough to render the unintended loss of consciousness unlikely.'

The two aspects of patient communication and drugs with wide safety margins remain the greatest asset of safe conscious sedation.

It was not until 1990 and the appearance of the Poswillo Report that the situation changed significantly. In his report, Poswillo amended the definition of simple conscious sedation to: 'A carefully controlled technique in which a single intravenous drug, or a combination of oxygen and nitrous oxide, is used to reinforce hypnotic suggestion and reassurance in a way which allows dental treatment to be performed with minimal physiological and psychological stress, but which allows verbal contact with the patient to be maintained at all times. The technique must carry a margin of safety wide enough to render the unintended loss of consciousness unlikely. Any technique of sedation other than as defined above should be regarded as coming within the meaning of dental general anaesthesia.'

The use of a single drug (or nitrous oxide/oxygen) is ideally suited to most cases but the suggestion that all other techniques should be regarded as general anaesthetics did not find universal support. The most recent advice from the Joint Dental Faculties of the Royal College of Surgeons of England (1996) and the current advice from the General Dental Council, published in late 1997, adopt a definition largely identical to the original one of John Wylie.

In terms of clinical advancement, recent developments in sedation have focused on the possibility of using patient-controlled administration and the use of propofol. This inert phenol derivative is an excellent, short-acting intravenous anaesthetic agent which in theory should suffer from all the objections raised in the administration of intermittent methohexitone. However, the advent of patient-controlled analgesia in postoperative pain control following surgery has raised the possibility that similar machines could be adapted for use in the dental surgery. Whether they will ever be appropriate for use by a single operator-sedationist in a general practice setting remains to be seen.

The other area of development centres on the possibilities of reversible sedation. Modern general anaesthesia relies heavily on such techniques and they have proved extremely effective in regulating anaesthetic depth and duration. It seems logical that modern sedation should be able to expect the development of similar techniques and the introduction of flumazenil (Anexate®) represents a potential first step along this route.

It is certain that further innovation will occur. There is much to be gained from the practice of safe conscious sedation, not just in dentistry but in many other areas of surgery. As with the history of anaesthesia, dentistry has taken the opportunity to lead the way thus far and to point to the ongoing possibilities of further development. This must be based on a sound understanding of the principles and practice of safe sedation and the remainder of this book aims to give such a grounding.

References and further reading

Ajzen, I. and Fishbein, M. (1989). *Understanding Attitudes and Predicting Social Behaviour.* New Jersey: Prentice Hall.

Chaves, J.F. (1997). Hypnosis in dentistry; historical overview and current appraisal. In *Hypnosis in Dentistry* (M. Mehrstedt and P. Wilkstrom, eds). Munich: Stiftung.

Crawford, A.N. (1997). A dental support group for anxious patients. *Br. Dent J.*, **183**, 57–62.

Department of Health (1990). Report of an Expert Working Party on General Anaesthesia, Sedation and Resuscitation in Dentistry. London: HMSO.

General Dental Council (1997). Maintaining Standards: Guidance to Dentists on Professional and Personal Conduct. London: General Dental Council.

Hayes, N. (1994). *Foundations of Psychology; An Introductory Text.* London: Routledge.

Royal College of Surgeons of England (1993). Guidelines for sedation by non-anaesthetists. Report of a Joint Working Party.

Royal College of Surgeons of England (1996). *Report of the Joint Dental Faculties Working Party on Sedation.* London: Royal College of Surgeons of England.

Todd, J.E. and Lader, D. (1991). *Adult Dental Health; 1988.* London: HMSO.

2

Applied anatomy and physiology

Introduction

An integrated approach to the anatomy, physiology and to some extent the pharmacokinetics of the drugs as they relate to sedation is essential to establish a basis for safe clinical practice (the actual pharmacology of the individual agents used for sedation is to be found in Chapter 4). This chapter deals principally with the application of these subjects, rather than simply repeating details that could easily be found in the various textbooks of anatomy, physiology or pharmacology. It is, however, the authors' experience that students frequently fail to grasp the basics of these subjects in the early parts of their courses because they fail to see how they relate to clinical practice. Sound clinical practice must be based on a solid foundation of basic medical science and the following sections address the relevant anatomy, physiology and general pharmacokinetics of sedation.

The action of a sedative

All sedatives produce their effects by acting on the brain. This applies to gaseous, oral and intravenous agents although their exact modes of action may differ. The mode of action of a drug is referred to as its pharmacodynamics and these are the results caused by the activity of the drug on the central nervous system. They are essentially the same whether a drug is given orally, intravenously or by inhalation. Drugs which are given orally have to be absorbed from the gut and whilst some drugs are absorbed in part from the stomach most absorption occurs from the intestines. This is affected by the physical processes of digestion and the absorption profile of the drugs which are subject to considerable individual variation. With an intravenous agent, the drug is introduced directly into the blood stream by injection rather than via the gut or the lungs and this will be considered below in the section about intravenous drugs and excretion. With an inhalational agent, the gas must enter the lungs, cross the alveolar membranes to be absorbed into the blood, be pumped around the left side of the heart into the arterial blood before reaching the tissues of the body. There are, therefore, three aspects of this process: entry into the lungs; circulation to the tissues, and excretion or removal from the body.

Lung entry

Inhalational agents can be either gaseous or vaporized. Vapours are essentially in liquid form at room temperature and have to be mixed with a gas by controlled evaporation or 'vaporization'. Vapours are, therefore, usually expressed in terms of a percentage of the carrier gases whereas the gases themselves are referred to as percentages of the whole mixture. In real terms the difference is insignificant since the percentage of a vapour is usually very small. Since higher percentages usually result in more profound effects (i.e. general anaesthesia), the use of vapours in inhalational sedation has really only been used on an experimental basis.

The effect of a gas (i.e. its degree of activity or depth of sedation) depends on several factors but the speed of onset is principally dependent on its partial pressure at the site of action. Partial pressure may be thought of as the force with which a gas is trying to come out of a solution in which it has been dissolved. In general terms it is inversely proportional to the solubility of a gas. Thus, nitrous oxide which has a very low solubility results in a rapid rise in partial pressure. The halogenated vapours (e.g. ethrane, isoflurane) have much higher solubilities and therefore respond with much slower rises in partial pressure.

The importance of understanding this cannot be emphasized enough since it affects both the potency of the gas or vapour and its speed of action. The less soluble gases or vapours are normally less potent but quicker acting. For this reason, a relatively insoluble gas like nitrous oxide is ideal for use in sedation since it combines two of the ideal properties for an inhalational agent, i.e. it is quick acting but not over potent. By virtue of its mode of action it is dependent on the process of respiration for initial entry into the lungs and some understanding of the process of respiration is essential.

Respiration is controlled by several groups of neurones, situated in the brain stem and collectively termed the 'respiratory centre'. This control centre receives information from a variety of sources including other brain receptors, the lungs, the blood vessels and the respiratory muscles (Figure 2.1). In addition, the respiratory centre receives information from various chemoreceptors in the medulla which monitor the pH of the cerebrospinal fluid. Changes in pH are largely influenced by the rise and fall of carbon dioxide levels since increased carbon dioxide availability leads to an increase in hydrogen ion availability as carbonic acid forms.

$$CO_2 + H_2O = H_2CO_3 = H^+ + HCO_3^-$$

In healthy individuals, the respiratory centre is thus able to provide very rapid responses to changes in pH or, in effect, $PaCO_2$ which it represents. Indeed, a rise of only 1 mmHg in the $PaCO_2$ will result in an increase in the ventilation rate of about 2.5 litres/minute. However, long term exposure of the chemoreceptors to chronically high $PaCO_2$ levels results in a diminished response and would be seen for instance in patients suffering from chronic bronchitis.

There are, in addition, chemoreceptors of a different type within the carotid bodies and these are generously supplied with arterial blood. They respond to falls in oxygen saturation (PaO_2) but their effect on the respiration rate is far less dramatic than that of the CO_2 receptors since they require a fall of nearly 50% of the PaO_2 before they have a clinically significant effect on the respiration rate.

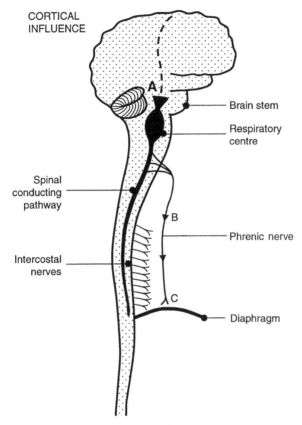

Figure 2.1 The control of respiration is influenced at several points. At point A, the respiratory centre is affected by all modern sedatives. At points B and C, the phrenic nerve and neuromuscular junction respectively, the influences are less profound than would be the case with general anaesthesia.

Information for the respiratory centre is also derived from stretch receptors in the lungs and respiratory muscles. All this information is used to process the control of breathing depth for regular breathing. Complex mechanisms (e.g. sneezing, coughing) are initiated by different receptors in the respiratory tract mucosa.

Finally, there is some control of breathing in the higher centres and indeed, control of breathing can be made a voluntary action—a feature which is used in some relaxation techniques. Normally, however, breathing and the processes of respiration occur involuntarily and, if fear or emotion threaten to make them too irregular, some attempt at voluntary control can be made.

Having processed the information from the chemoreceptors in the medulla, those in the carotid bodies and the information from the tactile receptors in the diaphragm, the process of breathing is initiated along the phrenic nerve. In normal breathing this involves contraction and relaxation of the diaphragm. Combined with the contraction of the intercostal muscles the rib cage is pulled upwards and outwards. This increases the internal volume of the thorax and thus creates a sub-atmospheric pressure which draws air in through the nose and/or mouth, past the pharynx, larynx and trachea to the bronchi. The bronchi comprise multiple bronchioles and alveoli—clusters of capillary-lined tissue which allow the perfusion of gases. The whole of this section of the respiratory process is termed inspiration.

In the reverse process (expiration), the diaphragm and intercostal muscles relax and the rib cage returns passively to its original shape. The alveolar blood, previously rich in carbon dioxide has moved on and the diffusion of carbon dioxide out of the blood and the loss of oxygen from the inspired air results in a gas mixture containing some 5% carbon dioxide and only 16% oxygen; the nitrogen content remains virtually constant. The processes of inspiration and expiration comprise the process of external respiration. Inspiration is a highly muscular process whilst expiration is relatively passive, thus explaining why people with asthma (bronchial spasm) find breathing out much harder than breathing in when they are suffering an attack.

If there is obstruction of the upper airway, this may result in 'paradoxical respiration'. Paradoxical or 'see-saw' respiration is the result of the diaphragm and intercostal muscles contracting in an attempt to increase the size of the thorax. When this does not occur (due to the obstruction) the dimensions actually decrease whilst the abdominal volume increases. As this is the exact reverse of what would be anticipated during the inspiratory phase (and as the exact opposite also occurs in the expiratory phase) the term 'paradoxical' respiration is used.

Assuming that there is no obstruction and normal breathing ensues, a healthy adult will inspire and expire about 450 ml of air each breath—a figure known as the tidal volume. In the course of a minute, about 12 breaths would be taken—known as the respiration rate. This allows the calculation of the minute volume which can be expressed as:

$$\text{MINUTE VOLUME} = \text{TIDAL VOLUME} \times \text{RESPIRATION RATE}$$

A simple calculation (450 ml $\times$ 12) shows this to be just over 5 litres per minute in a healthy adult although allowances need to be made for size and other factors. Of that volume only two-thirds ever reaches the alveoli of the lungs where it is available for gas transfer. The remaining part, occupying the nose, pharynx, trachea and bronchi, which is not available for gas transfer, is known as the dead space. This needs to be borne in mind when designing inhalational sedation equipment since badly designed machinery and tubing can significantly increase the dead space.

Circulation to the tissues

As mentioned earlier an inhalational agent must enter the lungs and cross the alveolar membranes to be absorbed into the blood (the processes relating to intravenous agents will be considered in the next section). During the induction of sedation each breath of nitrous oxide results in a small but incremental rise in the partial pressure. Partial pressure is dependent on the solubility (or lack thereof) of the gas and this is expressed as the blood–gas coefficient. Blood–gas or partition coefficient is defined as the ratio of the number of molecules of a gas in the blood phase to the number of molecules in the gaseous phase at a point of equilibrium. Soluble agents have higher values (e.g. ether is about 13) whilst gases of low solubility have low values (e.g. nitrous oxide is 0.47).

As the nitrous oxide dissolves in the alveolar blood it is rapidly transported away via the pulmonary vein to the left side of the heart. It is then ejected into the circulation though the aorta and thence via the arteries and arterioles to the capillary blood vessels where gas exchange with the tissues takes place (see below for details of the functional anatomy). The speed of this process is dependent on the cardiac output—the volume of blood ejected into the circulation each minute from the left ventricle. If the cardiac output is high, a relatively large volume of blood also flows through the lungs. This means that the same amount of gas (i.e. each tidal volume) is taken into a larger volume of blood resulting in a lower concentration (concentration = mass per unit volume). Conversely, patients with a lower cardiac output have less blood available for gas diffusion and therefore respond with a more rapid rise in partial pressure. This helps to explain why nitrous oxide is most effective when used to reinforce suggestion and when prior relaxation has helped to reduce heart rate and thus cardiac output. This also has a direct effect in reducing the patient's blood pressure since this is a factor of cardiac output and peripheral vascular resistance. There is some debate about what constitutes a 'safe' blood pressure but the greatest danger in this regard tends to be with sudden and unexpected changes, rather than the actual values a patient registers (see Chapter 3).

Whilst the processes of inspiration and expiration comprise external respiration (the means by which oxygen and carbon dioxide are interchanged in the lungs) it is the process of internal respiration (the means by which oxygen and carbon dioxide are interchanged in the tissues) which is perhaps most significant. In this respect, oxygen is of fundamental importance since the production of adenosine triphosphate (ATP) runs much more efficiently and for much longer when supplied with oxygen (aerobic metabolism) than when oxygen is not available or in short supply and anaerobic respiration has to occur.

An understanding of the passage of oxygen into and out of the bloodstream can be derived from consideration of partial pressures. Atmospheric pressure is usually between 750 and 770 mmHg or approximately 100 kilopascals (actually 752 mmHg = 100 kPa). Oxygen comprises nearly 21% of the atmospheric volume and so has a partial pressure of 21 kPa as it enters the nose.

In the lungs the presence of water vapour lowers the partial pressure of the oxygen by about 5% to just under 20 kPa. Since blood will saturate with an oxygen partial pressure of 16 kPa (120 mmHg), this is more than adequate to create a sufficient gradient across which the oxygen can diffuse into the blood—principally the haemoglobin of the red blood cells. The gradient must exist, however, since the oxygen does not get 'sucked' into the blood. The circulating venous blood has a residual oxygen content represented by a partial pressure of about 5–6 kPa (40 mmHg). After saturation, this level (i.e. the arterial PaO_2) increases to 13 kPa in a process known as arterialization.

Within the tissues the oxygen saturation varies, some organs being oxygen rich (e.g. liver, muscles at rest) and some relatively low (e.g. fat). Oxygen therefore leaves the blood when the pressure gradient is negative and enters the blood when it is positive.

The relationship between PaO_2 and haemoglobin saturation is well known as a dissociation curve (Figure 2.2) and can be influenced by a variety of factors. Shifts to the left result in lower availability of oxygen to the tissues; shifts to the

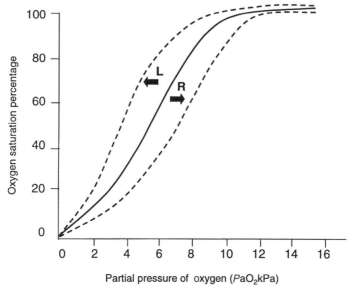

Figure 2.2 The oxygen/haemoglobin dissociation curve. The curve can be displaced to the left or the right by systemic influences which must be accounted for in seriously ill patients.

right increase the availability. An understanding of the significance of the S-shaped dissociation curve is also important since, like a car rolling down an incline, the pace of acceleration (i.e. desaturation) increases rapidly as the gradient increases. Fortunately, the converse is also true and re-oxygenation also occurs rapidly once the flow of oxygen to the lungs is established.

In the healthy adult every gram of haemoglobin is capable of absorbing nearly 1.4 ml of oxygen. Some simple maths enables the total volume of oxygen in the blood to be calculated but a small allowance must also be made for the oxygen dissolved in plasma (about 3 ml per litre). The concept of oxygen availability is important in all aspects of sedation, both inhalational and intravenous, and is summarized in Figure 2.3.

Anatomy of the cardiovascular system
The cardiovascular system is a complex, closed, body system which maintains the internal body environment in a situation of balance (homeostasis). The basic anatomy of the system with the heart, arteries, veins and capillaries is probably known to most schoolchildren and yet the anatomical distribution of the various

OXYGEN AVAILABILITY = ARTERIAL OXYGEN CONTENT × CARDIAC OUTPUT

ARTERIAL OXYGEN CONTENT = PLASMA OXYGEN + HAEMOGLOBIN OXYGEN

PLASMA OXYGEN CONTENT = 3 ml/l AT 37° AND 13 kPa

HAEMOGLOBIN OXYGEN CONTENT = HAEMOGLOBIN CONCENTRATION × 1.39 × % SATURATION

Figure 2.3 Oxygen availability is an important concept to bear in mind. The principles involved are illustrated in this figure.

veins and arteries can be both inconsistent and problematical. In addition, the physiological changes that occur within the vessels both in terms of their change in constituents (see above) and in the flow characteristics of the blood result in considerable variation in function.

The basic structure of the vessel wall is similar in all blood vessels with the tunica intima or endothelium lining the vessel's lumen. Externally is a connective tissue, the tunica adventitia which is slightly thicker in arteries. The middle layer is a layer of smooth muscle—the tunica media—which is much thicker in arteries and which is largely responsible for the peripheral control of blood pressure. The endothelial lining of veins is enveloped to form valves which, with externally muscular influence, assist in propelling blood back to the heart (valves are rarely taken into consideration during venepuncture, but they can be used to benefit or to hinder successful cannulation of a vein).

Blood returns to the right atrium via the venae cavae and is ejected from the right ventricle into the pulmonary circulation. The actual beating of the heart is initiated in the sino-atrial node and passes to the atrioventricular node along the Bundle of His. Innervation of the heart is influenced by the vagus nerve (X cranial/parasympathetic), through the nodes and also by sympathetic β_1 receptors which are situated throughout the heart walls. The vagus nerve stimulates a release of acetylcholine and this has the effect of slowing the heart whilst the sympathetic neurones release noradrenaline which increases both the rate and strength of contraction.

As well as the nervous and chemical stimulation, there are hormonal influences on the cardiovascular system. The kidneys produce renin which converts to angiotensin II which is an extremely powerful vasoconstrictor. In addition, the adrenal medulla can produce central release of catecholamines which simulate the action of the β receptors and induce sympathetic stimulation of the heart. Finally, there is a hormone released by the vessel endothelium known as endothelium derived relaxing factor (EDRF) and this causes vasodilatation.

Thus control of the cardiovascular system can be seen to consist of a highly complex series of mechanisms that can easily be disturbed by external factors such as sedation. In young and healthy individuals the compensatory mechanisms are more than adequate to deal with this but in the frail and elderly cardiovascular problems develop much more readily and allowance should always be made for this. This may also be true for those recovering from serious illnesses or who may be debilitated for any other reason.

Intravenous drugs and excretion

The vast majority of intravenous drugs are, after injection into the blood stream, carried in the blood plasma. Very few drugs bind to the blood cells in the way that oxygen does, for example. The plasma level (or concentration) causes the same type of diffusion gradient, however, to that described earlier with nitrous oxide and oxygen. This results in the drug crossing the tissue (or lipid) membranes to the site of action in the brain (it should be noted, of course, that the drugs cross other lipid membranes and not solely those in the brain!).

When a drug is injected it is present in the plasma in its manufactured form, i.e. dissolved in water or some other solvent. The drug may be ionized or un-ionized but drugs cannot penetrate lipid membranes in their ionized state. Only un-ionized drugs are lipid-soluble and only lipid-soluble drugs can penetrate lipid membranes. A drug may also be bound to a plasma protein when it also becomes ineffective at the site of action. An injected drug may therefore be free but ionized, bound to plasma proteins or free and un-ionized but only the last category will be effective. However, there is free interchange between the various states and this can have a dramatic effect on the mode and duration of action of a drug (see Figure 4.5).

Once circulating in the blood, a process of balancing the diffusion gradients occurs and this is generally referred to as redistribution—the passage of un-ionized lipid-soluble unbound drug into body tissues, mainly fat. This process largely explains the principle of the alpha half-life—$t_{1/2}\alpha$—which is the time taken for the serum concentration to fall by 50%. The $t_{1/2}\alpha$ is a useful clinical concept since it refers to the observed effects in a patient. Once a drug has been redistributed to the extent that its serum concentration has fallen below a therapeutic level the effect of the drug appears to have worn off. However, this must never be confused with the drug's $t_{1/2}\beta$ (the β or elimination half-life) which reflects the time it takes to remove half the drug from the body. The more quickly a drug is metabolized, the more the two half-lives appear similar.

The onset of action of an intravenous drug is dependent on four factors, two of which are the same as for the inhalational agents. These are:

1. The total dose injected—greater plasma levels obviously being achieved with higher doses.
2. The duration of injection—a shorter injection time resulting in a higher plasma level.
3. The cardiac output—see earlier.
4. The circulating blood volume—as would be expected, smaller blood volumes result in higher concentrations.

Recovery is also affected by the last two factors but principally by:

1. The rate and extent of redistribution of the drug within the tissues.
2. The rate and extent of liver metabolism.
3. The rate and extent of excretion.

With intravenous agents which are all highly lipid soluble, despite the less than generous blood supply to the adipose tissue compared with the brain or liver, the sheer mass of fat causes an increasing amount of the drug to be taken into the adipose tissues. This subsequently causes a reversal of the blood to brain diffusion gradient moving the drug back from the brain into the blood. Once the plasma concentration drops below the therapeutic level the patient begins to recover.

It cannot be stressed enough, however, that this does not represent a point at which the drug has left the body—a fact which may have dire consequences if further increments of a drug are added without allowing for the already circulating drug volume.

This has two potential effects. First, the dose of any increment required is likely to be considerably less than may have been expected and second, because of the reduced pressure gradients already present between the plasma and the tissues, recovery would be more prolonged than anticipated.

Recovery from a drug is therefore dependent on two physiological processes. Redistribution of the drug may allow clinical recovery from a drug's effects but metabolism (and excretion) is essential to remove the drug from the body's tissues. These two factors partly determine the profiles of a drug's action—its pharmacokinetics—whilst the actual mechanisms by which a drug actually works, i.e. what it does, are referred to as its pharmacodynamics. The details of these processes vary considerably with different drugs and largely determine the properties of an agent.

Drugs which circulate in the plasma are at some stage removed from the body and this process can occur in a variety of ways. With a relatively insoluble gas such as nitrous oxide, the gas is expelled rather than excreted. Some intravenous drugs too are expelled via the urine having been filtered out by the kidneys in their ionized or un-ionized state.

More commonly drugs are metabolized in the liver producing breakdown products known as metabolites. Some of these are themselves active drugs and, unless they are passed into the bile and not reabsorbed, they may produce secondary effects (as will be seen later this is a well known feature of some of the benzodiazepines). Normally the metabolites produced by the liver are delivered back into the plasma where they again pass via several diffusion gradients to the kidneys for excretion. It is only when a drug and all its metabolites have been completely cleared from the body that total recovery can be said to be complete. In some cases this may take days or occasionally even weeks to occur despite an agent appearing to be effective clinically for perhaps only a few hours. Thus, the importance of understanding the relationship between the anatomical and physiological function and the pharmacokinetics of a drug can be seen to be more important than just mere theory.

References and further reading

Atkinson, R.S., Rushman, G.B. and Davies, N.L.J. (1993). *Lee's Synopsis of Anaesthesia*, 11th edn. London: Butterworth Heinemann.

Emslie-Smith, D., Paterson, C.R., Scratcherd, T. and Read, N.W. (eds) (1988). *Textbook of Physiology*, 5th edn. Edinburgh: Churchill Livingstone.

Kelman, G.R. (1977). *Applied Cardiovascular Physiology*, 2nd edn. London: Butterworths.

Snell, R.S. (1995). *Clinical Anatomy for Medical Students*, 5th edn. Boston: Little, Brown.

3

Patient assessment

Introduction

Patient selection and assessment is an essential prerequisite to the success of subsequent treatment under conscious sedation. Careful pre-sedation appraisal will optimize the safety and effectiveness of sedation. The assessment is used to gain information from the patient in order to determine suitability for both sedation and dental treatment. It is also an opportunity for the patient to appraise and gain confidence in the clinician and for both to establish a mutual rapport. This is of particular importance for severely anxious and phobic dental patients who have often been put off dentistry by bad experiences in the past. Such patients need to be managed with care and reassurance in order to regain their trust and co-operation.

Whenever possible, pre-operative assessment should be undertaken at a specific appointment, on a separate day from that of the proposed treatment. The first meeting should ideally be away from the surgery environment, in a room which is not too 'clinical'. A relaxed demeanour will help to reassure the patient but it is important that the dental surgeon ensures that all the information required is obtained, both accurately and in sufficient detail. The accepted sequence of history taking, followed by examination, is no different from the assessment of any patient, but there should be special emphasis on the reasons for treatment under sedation and the patient's fitness to receive sedation. Only when all this information is available can an individual treatment plan be formulated. It is also important to gain indirect information about patients from the way they respond to questioning and, even more importantly, from the initial examination.

History

The history must include details of the nature of the patient's fear and anxiety, the past dental history and current dental symptoms, a thorough medical history and information on social circumstances. The medical history is the most important part of the history and will be covered in some detail.

Reason for fear

It is important from the outset to determine the nature of the patients' fear and this was dealt with in Chapter 1. This is the main reason why they have come along for possible treatment under sedation. Some people are frightened of 'dentistry' as a whole, whilst others have a specific fear about 'things in the mouth' or 'the dental drill' or 'dental injections' or 'having a tooth pulled'. The underlying basis for many of these fear-provoking stimuli is frequently the fear of 'pain'. Unfortunately dentistry has always had a close association with pain and the possibility of pain-free dental treatment can be a very difficult concept for anxious patients to accept.

The extent of dental anxiety can range from mild apprehension to true phobia. The phobic patient who presents with a poor dentition for routine conservation is very different from the patient who has an excellent dentition but is anxious about undergoing third molar surgery. It is important to try and gauge the degree of fear and it can be useful to ask the patient to complete a simple anxiety questionnaire which seeks information about their fears (Figure 3.1). This can help to break the ice and will steer the discussion in the right direction without unduly provoking sensitive emotions. In the case of fear of 'injections' or 'needles' the patient must be asked if this is a general fear or just specific to dentistry. Many patients have a fear of oral injections but will accept an injection in the arm. Clearly a complete true needle phobia will contra-indicate the use of intravenous sedation without some form of oral premedication.

Dental history

A detailed knowledge of the past dental history is essential, not only for planning dental treatment, but also for determining suitability to receive treatment under sedation.

The dental history should ascertain details of when the patient first became fearful of dentistry. For many patients their fear started with a bad experience in childhood but for others the onset of their anxiety may have been more recent, for example, following a traumatic extraction. Patients frequently state that they were quite happy to receive routine treatment until a specific dentist hurt them during treatment, which subsequently made them anxious about re-attending.

Information should also be sought about when (or even if!) the patient last underwent routine dental treatment and the type of dentistry received. It is helpful to find out whether the patient has received sedation previously and to ascertain their feelings about it. Finally, patients should be questioned about their concerns regarding their teeth, how they feel about their health and the appearance of their dentition, their future aspirations and any current dental symptoms. All of this information should then be compiled and used for treatment planning.

Medical history

A full medical history should be taken in the same way as for any patient presenting for dental treatment but special note should be made of cardiovascular, respiratory, hepatic and renal disease. Full details of current drug therapy will alert the dentist to potential drug interactions and may reveal undisclosed

Name: Date:

What aspects of dental treatment are you particularly concerned about (please circle your response):

   Coming for an appointment?

   Sitting in a dental chair?

   Having a dental examination?

   Having an injection in your mouth?

   Having a tooth drilled?

   Having your teeth scaled?

   Having a tooth filled?

   Having a tooth taken out?

   Other type of treatment (please specify)   ....

How long has it been since you last received routing dental care? .... months/years

What type of treatment have you received in the past (please circle your response)

   Scaling

   Filling

   Tooth extraction

   Other (please specifiy)   ....

What type of anaesthesia have you previously received for dental treatment?

   Local anaesthetic injection in the mouth

   General anaesthetic (completely asleep)

   Sedation (partly asleep)

Was there any specific event which initiated your fear of dentistry? ....
....

Figure 3.1 Dental anxiety questionnaire.

conditions. Patients at the extremes of the age range, pregnant women and handicapped patients deserve special consideration in relation to sedation. A medical history questionnaire may be helpful to ensure that all areas are covered and can provide prompts for further questioning (Figure 3.2). The aim of medical history taking is to determine the fitness of the patient to undergo sedation and is the most important factor to consider during assessment.

Name: Date of birth:

Have you ever had:

    Heart trouble, heart murmurs, high blood pressure, or rheumatic fever?

    Chest trouble or shortness of breath?

    Jaundice, hepatitis or other liver disease?

    Sleeping disorders?

    Kidney problems

    Any serious illnesses or infectious diseases (including HIV/AIDS)?

    Any operations, investigations or hospital admissions?

    A general anaesthetic or sedation?

Are you suffering or have you suffered from:

    Diabetes?

    Asthma, hay fever or eczema?

    Fainting, blackouts or epilepsy?

If appropriate could you be pregnant?

Are you allergic to penicillin or any other drugs?

Are you taking any medicines, tablets, skin creams or drugs?

How much do you smoke per day?

How much do you drink per day?

Further details (please add anything of medical importance):

Patient's signature: Date:

Figure 3.2 Medical history questionnaire.

Assessment of fitness

Deciding whether a patient is medically fit to undergo sedation can be difficult because of the vast range of medical conditions. A useful means of estimating fitness for sedation is to use the classification system introduced by the American Society of Anesthesiologists (ASA). In this system patients are allocated to specific grades according to their medical status and operative (or sedation) risk. The classification uses five grades as follows:

ASA I   Normal healthy patients
ASA II   Patients with mild systemic disease
ASA III   Patients with severe systemic disease that is limiting but not inca-
           pacitating
ASA IV   Patients with incapacitating disease which is a constant threat to life
ASA V   Moribund patients not expected to live more than 24 h.

Patients in ASA class I are ideally suited to receive conscious sedation. They pose the lowest risk and can be safely treated in general dental practice. Nevertheless, the possibility of undiagnosed medical problems should always be borne in mind, even in apparently healthy patients. ASA class II patients have a mild systemic disease. Examples might include well-controlled asthma, diet-controlled diabetes or mild hypertension. In addition to the true ASA class II patients it is also wise to include in this group patients who have no systemic disease but are extremely nervous, significantly overweight, or over 65 years of age. Extremely nervous patients have high circulating levels of endogenous adrenaline and are more prone to complications during sedation. Obese patients may have a reduced respiratory capacity and older people are generally more sensitive to sedation agents and their physiological processes are slower. Patients of ASA class II present a higher risk but, with appropriate precautions, many are also suitable treatment under sedation in dental practice.

Individuals in ASA class III represent a group that presents a difficult choice as far as sedation is concerned. This group includes patients who have, for example, stable angina, well-controlled epilepsy, chronic bronchitis, congestive heart failure or well-controlled insulin-dependent diabetes. These patients have a severe but well-controlled systemic disease, which may limit normal activity but which is not incapacitating.

The use of sedation to reduce physiological and psychological stress can be very beneficial to this category of patients and may well reduce the risk of an acute exacerbation of the medical condition during dental treatment. However, such patients do present an increased risk and most of them should be referred to a specialist environment where extra support is available.

ASA class IV represents patients who have severe life-threatening systemic disease. Examples include patients who have had a recent myocardial infarction, uncontrolled diabetes, uncontrolled epilepsy or severe emphysema requiring oxygen therapy. People in this category must be treated in hospital where full medical and anaesthetic support is available.

For patients in ASA class V, who are moribund, only emergency treatment would ever be provided.

The ASA classification is not infallible, and there is some overlap between categories, but it does represent a relatively simple means of determining the risk of sedation. It can be difficult to classify patients with multiple conditions, for example an asthmatic patient who has well-controlled diabetes; in general terms it is better to advance a person into the higher ASA group as a safety precaution on the 'better safe than sorry' principle.

Relevance of specific medical conditions

In order to assess accurately and categorize the medical fitness of a patient for sedation the dental surgeon must have a clear understanding of specific pathological and physiological processes and their relevance to sedation practice.

Cardiovascular disease
Disease of the heart and circulatory system will affect a patient's fitness for treatment under sedation. In the western world a high proportion of the population suffer from ischaemic heart disease and have a history of angina or a myocardial infarct. Patients with other conditions such as valvular or congenital heart disease may also attend the dental surgeon. In some of these patients the stress associated with dental treatment may lead to high levels of circulating adrenaline. This in turn causes tachycardia and hypertension, thereby increasing the load on the heart. When the cardiac status is already compromised stress may induce an acute exacerbation of the medical condition. The classic example of this would be the patient with stress-induced angina, who is at increased risk from acute myocardial infarction.

Hypertension resulting from vascular or renal disease affects many people, especially with increasing age. The stress of treatment and the effects of the sedation agent can cause significant fluctuations in blood pressure. Patients with a blood pressure below 160/95 should be able to receive sedation safely in dental practice. If the blood pressure is above this level, referral for medical evaluation before sedation is essential. In this regard the diastolic reading is probably the more significant of the two values. As mentioned earlier, however, it is sudden changes in blood pressure that give rise to greater concern than the initial readings.

Although patients with cardiovascular disease benefit considerably from receiving treatment under sedation, they do present a special risk. Their limited ability to cope with stress increases the chance of an acute exacerbation of the disease during the sedation appointment. Many are also taking cardio-active medication which can interact with sedation agents.

Respiratory disease
Virtually all sedation agents cause some degree of respiratory depression and good respiratory function is essential for patients undergoing sedation. Healthy patients with a normal respiratory capacity are able to compensate for the mild depressive effects of sedation drugs. Patients with respiratory disease have less respiratory reserve and can easily become deoxygenated under sedation.

Asthma is a disease which is increasing in incidence, especially amongst children. Patients with well-controlled mild asthma can receive sedation in dental practice but it is important to be aware that the stress of treatment may make asthma worse and appropriate precautions should be taken. Asthmatic patients should be asked to take a dose of their normal bronchodilator immediately prior to commencing sedation and emergency drugs should be available in the case of an acute attack (see Chapter 8). If the asthma is severe, requiring oral steroids or hospitalization, then the patient should be referred for sedation in a hospital environment.

In chronic bronchitis and emphysema, respiratory capacity is also severely reduced and the stimulus to respiration can switch from a high carbon dioxide drive to a low oxygen drive. Great caution should be exercised when considering sedation for this group of patients. Not only will the sedation agent cause further respiratory depression but the use of supplemental oxygen is inadvisable as it may further inhibit respiratory drive and possibly cause hypnoea or apnoea.

Upper respiratory tract diseases present a relative contra-indication to specific types of sedation. Inhalational sedation obviously requires a patent nasal airway for gas delivery but it is important in intravenous sedation also that the patient has no airway blockage. Chronic nasal obstruction caused by, for example, a deviated septum is more problematical and inhalational techniques may prove impossible for physical reasons in such cases.

Hepatic and renal disorders

Liver and kidney diseases affect the metabolism and excretion of sedation drugs, especially those administered by the oral and intravenous routes. The normal pharmacokinetics of sedation agents are altered in hepatic and renal disease (see Chapter 2), so that in such patients there can be a variable and unpredictable response. Those who receive sedation will be more sensitive to the sedative drug, may more easily become over-sedated and will take longer to recover. Any patient with a suspected history of hepatic or renal disease should be thoroughly investigated by a physician and, if the disease process is active or has resulted in permanent loss of function, sedation should only be undertaken in a hospital environment.

Neurological disorders

There is a diverse range of diseases of the nervous system which can present problems with sedation. One of the most common conditions is epilepsy. Benzodiazepines, because of their anticonvulsant action, should reduce the incidence of an acute fit during treatment. However, in theory, sedation can mask the classical features of a grand mal fit and if a convulsion does occur it may be difficult to diagnose. Unconsciousness may be the only sign and the cause can be difficult to distinguish from other medical and sedation-related complications and emergencies. Sedation should be restricted for use in well-controlled epileptics and, where doubt exists, it should be undertaken in a specialist environment where appropriate facilities are available to deal with an acute convulsion.

Endocrine disease

Diabetes, adrenal insufficiency and thyroid problems are the endocrine disorders which are most likely to present problems in relation to sedation. Diabetics who are diet-controlled or treated with oral hypoglycaemic drugs pose minimally increased risk to sedation in dental practice. The main area of risk relates to insulin-dependent diabetics (particularly when the diabetes is unstable and the blood sugar levels fluctuate significantly), where pre-operative starvation can upset the stability of blood sugar levels. The risk of hypoglycaemia occurring during sedation means that all insulin-controlled diabetics requiring sedation should be referred to hospital.

Adrenal insufficiency can be potentially dangerous to a patient undergoing sedation. The response to stress is suppressed and there may be secondary hypertension or diabetes. Patients on long-term steroids may have similar problems as a result of adrenal suppression. These individuals are at considerable risk under sedation and should be referred for specialist care when additional steroid cover can be given.

Patients with thyroid disorders must be stabilized before undergoing sedation and any patient with active thyroid disease should always be referred to hospital. Hyperthyroidism can cause tachycardia or even atrial fibrillation whilst hypothyroidism produces bradycardia and mental handicap, both of which can cause complications under sedation.

Haematological disorders
Anaemia is a common disorder which varies in severity. Mild chronic anaemia, such as that occurring as a result of menstrual blood loss, does not present a problem to sedation in dental practice. However, sedation should be avoided in patients with a history of the more severe forms of anaemia, especially sickle cell anaemia and thalassaemia. Such patients are at severe risk if subjected to a reduced oxygen tension, which can occur during sedation as a result of respiratory depression, especially if the patient is over-sedated. It should also be noted that patients with anaemia are less likely to develop cyanosis (i.e. appear blue-purple) due to the fact that they have less haemoglobin to become deoxygenated. This is because cyanosis does not become clinically apparent until at least 5 g/dl of de-oxygenated haemoglobin is present in the blood. Fortunately, this does not affect the readings of the pulse oximeter.

Disorders of the blood clotting system present a risk in relation to haemostasis. Injections should be avoided where at all possible and thus intravenous sedation is not the first choice method of anxiolysis. Inhalational sedation with nitrous oxide is useful because it not only provides sedation but also produces some analgesia, which may obviate the need for dental local anaesthetic injections for simple conservative dentistry. All patients with bleeding disorders or those who are receiving anticoagulant therapy should be treated in hospital.

Drug therapy
Drugs are intended to have a specific effect on one or more systems or organs of the body, but they can and frequently do produce coincidental side effects. Certain medicines interact with sedation drugs and it is imperative that the dental surgeon finds out exactly what drugs a patient is taking and the diseases for which they have been prescribed. Each medicine must be checked for potential interaction with sedative agents. If the patient cannot remember which drugs they have been prescribed then the dental surgeon must contact their general medical practitioner for clarification. It is essential to emphasize to patients undergoing sedation that they should continue taking their normal medication, unless they have been told otherwise by their doctor.

Table 3.1 indicates some key groups of drugs which interact with the benzodiazepines (BDZs) although some of the reactions are more theoretical possibilities. Care should always be taken, however, to ensure that a patient is not unnecessarily put at risk.

There are few absolute contra-indications to sedation as a direct result of drug therapy. Normally the underlying medical condition will determine the ultimate fitness of a patient for treatment. If sedation is to go ahead then appropriate precautions must be taken to allow for potential drug interactions. If an enhanced sedative effect is expected then the technique should be altered to slow the titration rate, reduce the total dose of sedation drug and allow more time for recovery.

Table 3.1 Interactions of benzodiazepines (BDZs) with drug groups

Drug	Potential interaction
Alcohol	Enhanced sedative effect
Analgesics (opioid)	Enhanced sedative effect
Antibacterials	Erythromycin inhibits metabolism of midazolam
Antidepressants	Enhanced sedative effect
Anti-epileptics	BDZs reduce effect of some anti-epileptics
Antihistamines	Enhanced sedative effect
Antihypertensives	Enhanced hypotensive effect
Antipsychotics	Enhanced sedative effect
Anti-ulcer drugs	Cimetidine inhibits metabolism of BDZs

Patients who are drug addicts or who abuse drugs should not be treated under sedation. Sedation is difficult to achieve in these individuals and there are many unpredictable interactions that can occur with the abused drugs. If there is any doubt about potential drug interaction then the patient should be referred to a specialist environment for treatment.

Pregnancy
There are two main risks with providing sedation in pregnancy. First, the potential teratogenic and sedative effects of sedation drugs on the foetus. Secondly, the patient may have an atypical response to sedation as a result of altered metabolism from the additional demands of the foetus. For both of these reasons it is preferable to postpone sedation until after the birth. Emergency or essential treatment should be undertaken in a hospital environment, preferably in the second trimester.

Mental or physical handicap
Patients with learning difficulties present special problems. Sedation can help mildly handicapped patients to undergo routine dental treatment whilst avoiding the need for life-long reliance on general anaesthesia. Unfortunately the individual tolerance and response of mentally handicapped patients to sedation is very unpredictable and these patients are best managed in a specialist environment. In contrast, physically handicapped patients usually respond very well to sedation and can be treated in dental practice if physical restraints allow. The more severe physical handicaps will require the special facilities available in hospital.

Age
Children and the elderly present a special risk to sedation, even if they are otherwise healthy. The metabolic rates of infants and young children are much higher than those of adults and their build is much smaller. The pharmacological effect of sedation agents in children is very variable and if a complication occurs the child's condition can deteriorate very rapidly. Only inhalational sedation should be provided for children in dental practice. Intravenous sedation should only ever be undertaken in special circumstances and in a hospital environment.

In older people, the functioning of body systems becomes progressively less efficient. They are more susceptible to the effects of sedation agents and smaller doses being required to avoid over-sedation. There is an increased incidence of undiagnosed disease and elderly patients are less able to cope with undue stress.

Although biological age rather than chronological age is the significant factor, caution should be exercised in sedating any patient over the age of 65.

If there is any doubt about a patient's medical status then communication with the general medical practitioner and/or referral to a specialist for sedation and treatment is essential.

Importance of social circumstances

The final part of the history is to evaluate the domestic circumstances of the patient. These are especially relevant to sedation in dental practice. A responsible adult will be required to accompany the patient and the availability of suitable transport is essential. Additional responsibilities such as children or elderly parents may make it difficult for some patients to attend and to recover safely at home. Adults should be questioned regarding their smoking habits and alcohol consumption and general enquiries about their domestic circumstances should be made.

Clinical examination

Assessment of a patient for treatment under sedation should consist of a full clinical examination and an assessment of vital signs. Radiographs and other investigations should be obtained before the procedure whenever this is possible.

Oral examination

Some patients may allow a full oral examination, charting of the teeth and intra-oral radiography. Those presenting for specific oral surgical procedures will usually be amenable to a normal examination. However, patients with moderate to severe dental anxiety may only agree to a superficial visual inspection, without using a probe. If oral examination is not feasible the patient may instead be agreeable to extra-oral dental panoramic tomography.

The aim of oral examination in anxious patients is to judge the type and extent of dental treatment required. This will help the dental surgeon to decide on the number of visits required and determine whether the treatment can be performed under sedation. For the majority of patients, who have often not been to a dentist for years, initial treatment will usually involve a gross scale, a number of extractions and routine conservation.

Sufficient information can usually be gleaned from which to compile a treatment plan for the first sedation appointment. Examination of anxious dental patients requires some degree of compromise and occasionally full examination and intra-oral radiography will have to be postponed until a later date when the patient is sedated.

Assessment of vital signs

At the assessment appointment it is important to measure the heart rate, blood pressure, respiration rate and weight. The purpose of taking preliminary values is threefold:

1. To determine the patient's fitness for sedation.
2. To provide baselines for comparison with future measurements taken during sedation.
3. As a screening to reveal possible undiagnosed disease.

Some degree of elevation in the cardiorespiratory signs, such as tachycardia or systolic hypertension, above the normal range for the age and sex of the patient, is to be expected at the assessment appointment. This is caused by acute apprehension felt by anxious dental patients when they attend the dental surgery.

Blood pressure can be measured using either a manual or automatic sphygmomanometer (Figure 3.3). The blood pressure can be used to categorize a patient into an appropriate ASA class, as follows (based on Malemud, 1995):

Blood Pressure	ASA Class
Less than 140/90	I
From 140/90 to 159/94	II
From 160/95 to 199/114	III
Over 200/115	IV

As previously stated a patient with a blood pressure below 160/95 can be treated under sedation in dental practice. If the blood pressure is above this level, the patient should be referred to his/her general medical practitioner for full evaluation before considering sedation.

Although weight is recorded, the result is only of significance if the patient is very over- or under-weight. Weight is not used to calculate the dose of sedation drug because sedation is administered by titration. However, patients

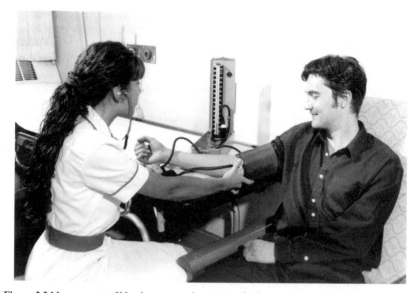

Figure 3.3 Measurement of blood pressure using a manual sphygmomanometer.

who are excessively obese should be treated with caution. If the Body Mass Index (weight in kg/height in m^2) is greater than 30, the patient will probably not be suitable for sedation in dental practice and should be referred to hospital. At the other end of the spectrum patients who have a very small build, especially children and the elderly, tend to be more susceptible to the effects of sedation.

Treatment planning

Armed with the detailed information from the history and examination, a preliminary treatment plan can now be established. This needs to specify both the type of sedation or anaesthesia plus the dental treatment required. It needs to be approached both logically and flexibly, allowing for modifications if they become necessary.

Choice of sedation technique

Although the aim of this chapter has focused on assessing the suitability of patients for sedation, it is important to remember the range of treatment options including:

1. Local analgesia alone.
2. Sedation and local analgesia.
3. General anaesthesia.

In considering the type of sedation or anaesthesia, account should be taken of the patient's medical fitness, social circumstances, degree of anxiety and expected level of co-operation, plus the extent and duration of the planned dental treatment. It is also important to establish the clinical need for the type of sedation or anaesthesia selected. Some patients, such as those with minimal anxiety, requiring relatively simple surgical extractions, may be agreeable to having treatment under local analgesia alone. Others may be so terrified because of their phobia or because they require traumatic or extensive dental procedures that general anaesthesia would be the best choice. In between these two extremes there are a large proportion of patients for whom techniques of pharmacological sedation represent the most acceptable means of undergoing dental treatment. Careful explanation and discussion of the different types of sedation with the patient is essential. The dental surgeon should describe the main features of oral, inhalational and intravenous techniques and point out the key differences between sedation and general anaesthesia. Many patients have the preconceived idea that they will only undergo treatment if they are completely 'asleep' or 'knocked out'. It is important to explain that sedation produces relaxation, decreased awareness and amnesia, but not unconsciousness. Reassurance should also be given about painless local anaesthetic administration and the use of topical analgesia.

All explanations must be carried out in a particularly considerate manner and the patient's reaction during the explanation is helpful in deciding the most appropriate sedation technique. Patients should also be reassured that they remain in control of their own destiny and that no treatment will be forced upon them against their wishes (see Chapter 9).

Dental treatment plan

Dental treatment planning for oral surgical patients is usually relatively straight-forward. However, for severely anxious and phobic dental patients the treatment plan depends on a number of factors. Their current dental condition, predicted future attendance pattern and compliance with oral health instructions should all be taken into account. The purpose of this is to provide good quality dentistry consistent with the patients' realistic aspirations. There is little point in doing molar endodontics or bridgework on patients who are unlikely to maintain their oral health in the long term. Treatment of teeth that are causing symptoms should be the first priority. This will be followed by extraction of retained roots and grossly carious or periodontally involved teeth. Gross scaling and simple, good quality conservation should be the mainstay of treatment for the remaining teeth. These are only general recommendations and it is essential that each patient has an individual treatment plan tailored to his/her own needs. The patient should be given an estimate of the number of appointments that will be required to complete the work and of the arrangements for long-term follow-up.

Preparation of patients for sedation

Patients who are scheduled to receive sedation must receive careful verbal and written instructions (Figure 3.4) as to their responsibilities before and after the sedation appointment.

For oral and intravenous sedation, the patient should be accompanied by a responsible adult. With inhalational sedation, this is a slightly controversial subject since there is good evidence that patients acquire their normal faculties within minutes of sedation being terminated. Escorts must accompany the patient to and from the dental practice and must assume responsibility for the patient's post-sedation care. Wherever possible the patient and escort should travel home by private car or taxi rather than by public transport. Patients should be warned against driving, operating machinery (including domestic appli-ances), drinking alcohol or signing legal documents for a period of 24 hours following sedation. It is recommended that patients are asked to starve for a period of 2 hours before the sedation appointment. Within 2–4 hours of sedation, patients should be advised to take a light meal with tea or fruit juice. Longer periods of starvation are not advisable as the relative hypoglycaemia that occurs during starvation may precipitate fainting during the sedation appoint-ment. Additionally, long periods of starvation result in acid build-up in the stomach and the risk of regurgitation rises with time in such cases. In an appropriately sedated patient the protective laryngeal reflexes are not obtunded and thus the risk of aspiration if the patient vomits should be minimal.

Written, informed consent must be obtained from all patients who are to receive treatment under sedation. The dental surgeon must carefully explain to the patient what to expect at the treatment appointment. This should include a description of the sedation technique and its side effects and detail of the dentistry to be provided. The patient should sign a consent form giving permis-sion not only for the sedation but also for the local analgesia and dental treatment. It is not best practice to leave obtaining consent until the day of treatment when the patient may be particularly anxious and unable to make clear

---

Patient Instruction Sheet

You have been offered sedation in order to help you relax. Most people find that this is a pleasant and acceptable way of receiving dental treatment. You will have the sedation agent administered either through an injection in the back of the hand (intravenous sedation) or via a small mask placed over your nose (inhalation sedation). Once you feel drowsy and sufficiently relaxed, your mouth will be numbed and the dental work will be commenced. During the procedure you will feel peaceful and largely unaware of what is going on; in fact many patients do not remember anything about their treatment. At the end of the session you will be allowed to recover until you are fit enough to be discharged home with your escort.

It is essential that you observe the following instructions, otherwise your sedation appointment may be cancelled.

1. You MUST NOT eat or drink anything for two hours prior to your appointment time. Before this you should have a light meal, e.g. toast and tea, coffee or fruit juice.

2. You MUST be accompanied by a responsible adult who must remain in the waiting room throughout your appointment, escort you home afterwards and arrange for you to be looked after for the following 24 hours.

3. If you are taking any medicines they should be taken at the usual times and should also be brought with you so that the dental surgeon may know what they contain.

4. Any illness occurring before the appointment should be reported immediately, as this may affect your treatment.

5. Your escort should take you home after treatment by private car rather than by public transport.

6. You MUST NOT drive any vehicle, operate any machinery or use any domestic appliance for 24 hours after sedation.

7. You MUST NOT drink alcohol, return to work, make any important decisions or sign any legal documents for 24 hours after sedation.

If you follow these instructions you will find your treatment under sedation both pleasant and uneventful. Please feel free at any time to ask the dental surgeon or nurse any questions that you may have about your treatment.

Figure 3.4 Written instruction sheet for patients scheduled for sedation.

judgements for valid consent. Equally, however, consent should be obtained within a reasonable period of time prior to the appointment for sedation.

Finally, any remaining questions that the patient has should be answered and an appointment should then be made to start treatment under sedation.

Assessment record

Full details of the history, examination and treatment plan must be recorded in the patient notes. It is also useful to complete a sedation assessment form, an example of which is shown in Figure 3.5. Use of a standardised form ensures that all aspects of the assessment are covered and also provides a readily

SEDATION ASSESSMENT

Patients Name		Date of Birth	Record Number

Assessment Date	Assessed by

Social History	Relevant Details
Age/Occupation	
Smoking/Alcohol	

Medical Conditions	Relevant Details
Cardiovascular disease	
Respiratory disease	
Hepatic/Renal disease	
Bleeding/Epilepsy/Diabetes	
Anaemia/Jaundice/Hepatitis	
Other Serious Illness	
Operations/GA/Sedation	
Drug Therapy	
Drugs/Medications	
Allergies	

Vital Signs				ASA Class
Weight	Blood Pressure	Pulse	Respiration Rate	

Treatment Plan	
Type of Sedation (IV/RA/Oral)	
Dental treatment plan - 1	
- 2	
- 3	
Written consent	
Written information & instructions	
Date of treatment appt	

Signature of dental surgeon	

Figure 3.5 Sedation assessment form.

accessible summary which can be referred to at the treatment appointment. If all the documentation is correctly completed, the likelihood of accidents is reduced and the defence of any accusations facilitated!

References and further reading

Berggren, U. and Meynert, G. (1984). Dental fear and avoidance: causes, symptoms and consequences. *Journal of the American Dental Association*, **109**, 247–251.

Malemud, S.F. (1995). *Sedation: a Guide to Patient Management*. St Louis: Mosby, pp. 32–62.

Ryder, W. and Wright, P.A. (1988). Dental sedation: a review. *British Dental Journal*, **165**, 207–215.

Skelly, A.M. (1992). Sedation in dental practice. *Dental Update*, **19**, 61–67.

4

Pharmacology of inhalation and intravenous sedation

Introduction

A sound understanding of the principles of pharmacokinetics and of the individual sedation agents is essential to the safe practice of sedation. It is important from the outset to specify exactly what is meant by a sedation agent as there can be considerable overlap between drugs which produce both sedation and general anaesthesia. A drug used for sedation should:

1. Depress the central nervous system to an extent that allows operative treatment to be carried out with minimal physiological and psychological stress.
2. Modify the patient's state of mind such that communication is maintained and the patient will respond to verbal command.
3. Carry a margin of safety wide enough to render the unintended loss of consciousness and loss of protective reflexes unlikely.

Modern sedation practice should only use agents and techniques which satisfy the above criteria. Additionally, the agents themselves should have a:

1. simple method of administration;
2. rapid onset;
3. predictable action and duration;
4. rapid recovery;
5. rapid metabolism and excretion;
6. low incidence of side effects.

Sedation agents are usually administered via the inhalational, intravenous or oral routes. The route of administration affects the timing of drug action, although ultimately all drugs arrive at their target cells in the brain via the blood stream.

Inhalation agents have the advantage of being readily absorbed by the lungs to provide a rapid onset of sedation, followed by rapid elimination and recovery. Intravenous agents are predictably absorbed but once administered cannot be removed from the blood stream. The action of intravenous agents is terminated by re-distribution, metabolism and excretion. Oral sedatives have a less certain absorption due to variability of gastric emptying and they therefore produce unpredictable levels of sedation.

This chapter will primarily address the pharmacology of sedation agents currently used in inhalational and intravenous techniques and builds on the fundamental principles which were the subject of Chapter 2. The pharmacology of the oral sedatives will be covered in Chapter 7.

Inhalational sedation agents

Inhalational agents produce sedation by their action on various areas of the brain. They reach the brain by entering the lungs, crossing the alveolar membrane into the pulmonary veins, returning with the blood to the left side of the heart and then passing into the systemic arterial circulation. Thus the two main components of inhalational sedation are the entry of the inspired gas into the lungs and distribution of the agent by the circulation to the tissues.

Basic pharmacology of inhalational sedatives

The basic pharmacokinetics of sedation were discussed in Chapter 2 and are dealt with in this chapter in relation mainly to nitrous oxide, the principal inhalational sedative. During the induction of inhalational sedation, each breath containing nitrous oxide raises the partial pressure of the gas in the alveoli. As the alveolar partial pressure rises the gas is forced across the alveolar membrane into the blood stream, whence it is carried to the site of action in the brain. The gas passes down a pressure gradient from areas of high partial pressure to areas of low partial pressure (Figure 4.1). The level of sedation is proportional to the partial pressure of the agent at the site of action. After termination of gas administration the reverse process occurs. The partial pressure in the alveoli falls and the nitrous oxide passes in the opposite direction out of the brain, into the circulation and thence into the lungs.

The rate at which a gas passes down its pressure gradient is determined by its solubility. The solubility of a sedation agent (i.e. the blood–gas partition

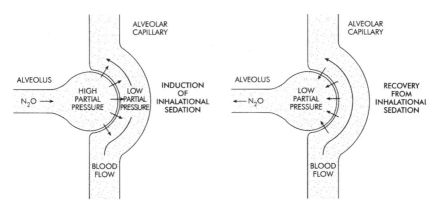

Figure 4.1 Movement of nitrous oxide gas down the partial pressure gradient during induction and recovery from inhalational sedation.

coefficient, see Chapter 2) determines how quickly the partial pressure in the blood and ultimately the brain will rise or fall. The higher the partition coefficient, the greater the alveolar concentration of the agent needs to be in order to produce a rise in partial pressure in the blood and ultimately the tissues. For the purposes of sedation, a gas with a low partition coefficient is preferred. Small concentrations of gas will produce a rapid rise in partial pressure and a fast onset of sedation. Similarly, after cessation of gas administration there will be a rapid fall in partial pressure and a fast recovery. It is the inspired concentration of sedation agent which will determine the final level of sedation. The speed of induction of sedation is influenced by the rate of increase in gas concentration, and the minute volume and cardiac output of the patient (Figure 4.2). Any increase in minute volume, such as can be caused by asking the patient to take deep breaths, will increase the speed of onset of sedation. Conversely, an increase in cardiac output will reduce the speed of induction of sedation. With a high cardiac output there is an increased volume of blood passing through the lungs. The sedation agent present in the lungs will be taken up into this larger volume of blood and the actual concentration of gas transported per unit volume of blood will be lower. Thus less sedation agent will reach the brain and there will be a slower onset of sedation. The speed of recovery after termination of gas administration is similarly affected by the same factors.

Potency of inhalational sedation agents

All sedation agents will produce general anaesthesia if used in high enough doses. The key to modern sedation practice is to ensure that the agents used have a wide enough margin of safety to render the unintended loss of consciousness unlikely. This means that there should be a considerable difference in the dose required to produce a state of sedation and the dose needed to induce general anaesthesia.

For inhalational anaesthetic agents the potency is expressed in terms of a 'minimum alveolar concentration' (MAC). The MAC of an agent is the inspired concentration which will, at equilibrium, abolish the response to a standard surgical stimulus in 50% of patients. Although the inspired concentration is measured as a percentage, the MAC is usually expressed as a number. Equilibrium is achieved when the tissue concentration of the gas equals the inspired concentration. MAC is a useful index of potency and is used to compare different anaesthetic gases.

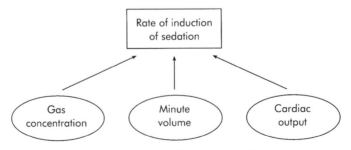

Figure 4.2 Factors influencing the rate of onset of inhalational sedation.

Gases used for sedation should preferably have a moderate or high MAC and a low solubility. This will ensure a broad margin of safety between the incremental doses used to produce sedation and the final concentration required to induce anaesthesia. It would be very easy, using an agent with a small MAC for sedation, to accidentally overdose and anaesthetise a patient.

Types of inhalational sedative

Nitrous oxide

Nitrous oxide is the only inhalational agent currently in routine use for conscious sedation in dental practice. The uninterrupted use of nitrous oxide as the basic constituent of gaseous anaesthesia for over 150 years following its discovery, demonstrates its acceptability and usefulness. In the 1930s, nitrous oxide was used for sedation purposes in the Scandinavian countries, particularly Denmark. However, it was not until the 1960s, when Harold Langa from the United States expounded the modern practice of relative analgesia, that nitrous oxide came into widespread use as a sedation agent in dentistry.

Nitrous oxide is a colourless and virtually odourless gas with a faintly sweet smell. It is heavier than air with a specific gravity of 1.53 and is stored in light blue cylinders in liquid form at a pressure of 750 pounds per square inch (43.5 bar). The gas is sold by weight and each cylinder is stamped with its empty weight. As the contents of the cylinder are liquid the pressure inside, as measured by the pressure gauge on the inhalational sedation machine, will remain constant until nearly all the liquid has evaporated. The value shown on the gauge does not decrease in a linear fashion and tends to fall rapidly immediately before the cylinder becomes empty. Thus the only reliable means of assessing the amount of nitrous oxide in a cylinder is to weigh the cylinder and to compare the value with the weight of the empty cylinder. It can also be tapped with a metal instrument by those with musical ears when the pitch of the note changes as the gas is used. In addition, after prolonged use, the evaporation of the liquid nitrous oxide causes ice crystallization on the cylinder at the level of the liquid within, thereby providing a third indication as to the nitrous oxide volume remaining in the cylinder.

Nitrous oxide has a low blood gas partition coefficient of 0.47, so it is relatively insoluble and produces rapid induction of sedation. A further consequence of the poor solubility is that when administration is discontinued, nitrous oxide dissolved in the blood is rapidly eliminated via the lungs. During the first few minutes of this elimination large volumes of nitrous oxide pour out of the blood and into the lungs. This can actually displace oxygen from the alveoli causing a condition known as diffusion hypoxia. This occurs because the volume of nitrous oxide in the alveoli is so high that the patient effectively 'breathes' 100% nitrous oxide. For this reason the patient should receive 100% oxygen for a period of 1–2 minutes after the termination of nitrous oxide sedation.

Nitrous oxide has a theoretical minimum alveolar concentration of 105. The high MAC means that that nitrous oxide is a weak anaesthetic which is readily titrated to produce sedation. Because the MAC is over 80, it is theoretically impossible to produce anaesthesia using nitrous oxide alone, at normal atmospheric pressure, in a patient who is adequately oxygenated. However, caution should be exercised when using inhaled concentrations of nitrous oxide over

50%, because even at this relatively low percentage some patients may enter a stage of light anaesthesia.

Nitrous oxide is a good sedation agent producing both a depressant and euphoriant effect on the central nervous system. It is also a fairly potent analgesic. A 50% inhaled concentration of nitrous oxide has been equated to that of parenteral morphine injection at a standard dose (10 mg in a 70-kg adult). It can be used to good effect to facilitate simple dentistry in patients who are averse to local analgesia and it decreases the pain of injections in those who require supplemental local anaesthesia. Nitrous oxide has few side effects in therapeutic use. It causes minor cardiorespiratory depression, is minimally metabolized and produces no useful amnesia.

The main problems associated with the use of nitrous oxide relate not to the patient but to the staff actually providing sedation and the potential hazards of chronic exposure to nitrous oxide gas have recently been recognized. It has been shown that regular exposure of health care personnel to low levels of nitrous oxide can cause specific illnesses, the most common effects being haematological disorders and reproductive problems (Figure 4.3). It is well known that nitrous oxide causes the oxidation of vitamin B_{12} and affects the functioning of the enzyme, methionine synthetase. This in turn impairs haematopoeisis and can give rise to pernicious anaemia in staff exposed to nitrous oxide for prolonged periods. Dental surgeons who have abused nitrous oxide have been shown to have the debilitating neurological signs of pernicious anaemia (Figure 4.4). There is a proven increase in the rate of miscarriages in female dental surgeons, dental nurses and, perhaps surprisingly, in the wives of male dental surgeons who have been exposed to nitrous oxide gas. Dental nurses assisting with nitrous oxide sedation are also twice as likely to suffer a miscarriage than other dental nurses. Nitrous oxide has also been shown to cause decreased female and male fertility. Each hour of exposure to unscavenged nitrous oxide leads to a 6% reduction in the probability of conception in each menstrual cycle. Other chronic effects of nitrous oxide exposure are much rarer but are said to include hepatic and renal disease, malignancy and cytotoxicity.

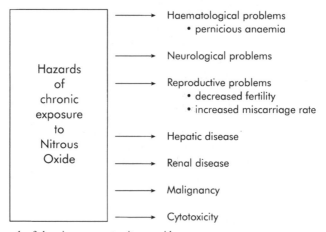

Figure 4.3 Hazards of chronic exposure to nitrous oxide.

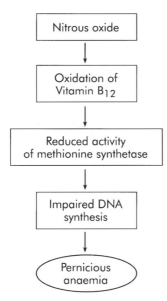

Figure 4.4 Effect of chronic nitrous oxide exposure on haematopoiesis. By oxidizing vitamin B_{12} and inhibiting the enzyme methionine synthetase, nitrous oxide inhibits DNA synthesis and produces the clinical features of pernicious anaemia.

The subject of nitrous oxide pollution has become a world-wide health and safety issue, particularly as it also appears to damage the ozone layer. Regulations now define the maximum acceptable occupational exposure of personnel to nitrous oxide, which in the UK should not average more than 100 p.p.m. over an 8-hour period under the current Health and Safety regulations. The risks to health care personnel working with nitrous oxide have been reduced considerably by the introduction of efficient scavenging and ventilation systems. If exhaled nitrous oxide is actively removed then there will be less pollution of the atmosphere where health care personnel are working.

Other inhalational agents
Volatile anaesthetic agents such as halothane and isoflurane have been tested for use in inhalational sedation. Unfortunately they are very potent drugs with low MAC values (the MAC of halothane is 0.76). This makes it difficult to titrate the drug concentration to produce sedation without exceeding the narrow margin of safety and inducing general anaesthesia. These drugs are not currently suitable for providing sedation in dental practice and do not comply with the basic definitions of safe sedation.

The role of oxygen

Oxygen is not a sedation agent. However, it is of such fundamental importance to inhalational sedation technique that it deserves further mention. Inhalational sedation agents are always delivered in an oxygen-rich mixture containing a minimum of 30% oxygen by volume. Oxygen is stored as a gas in black cylinders with white shoulders, at a pressure of 2000 pounds per square inch (137 bar). Because it is a gas under pressure, the gauge on the inhalational sedation machine will give an accurate representation of the amount of oxygen contained in the cylinder. The oxygen supply used for inhalational sedation should be separate from, and additional to, the supply kept for use in the management of emergencies. Oxygen will sustain and enhance combustion and therefore no naked flames should be allowed in an area where oxygen is being used. Mechanisms of oxygen uptake and transport were described in Chapter 2 and a grasp of their understanding is essential to the safe practice of sedation.

Intravenous sedation

Intravenous sedation agents are injected directly into the blood stream where they are carried in the plasma to the tissues. The plasma level of the sedative attained during injection causes the agent to diffuse down its concentration gradient across the lipid membranes to the site of action in the brain. The factors which influence the plasma level of the drug are therefore instrumental in determining the onset of action and recovery from the effect of the sedation agent.

As mentioned in Chapter 2, all drugs in the blood exist either free in the plasma or bound to plasma proteins. It is the free drug in its un-ionized form which provides the effective drug concentration (Figure 4.5). The plasma pH can affect the degree of dissociation of the drug into its ions. It is only the un-ionized free drug that is lipid soluble and able to penetrate the capillary membranes of the blood–brain barrier to reach the site of action in the brain. It is also the un-ionized fraction that is distributed into fat deposits and which undergoes metabolism in the liver. The relative movement between ionized and un-ionized forms is another factor affecting the pharmacokinetics of intravenous drugs.

Upon intravenous injection the plasma level of a sedation drug will rise rapidly. The agent will pass through the venous system to the right side of the heart and then via the pulmonary circulation to the left side of the heart. Once in

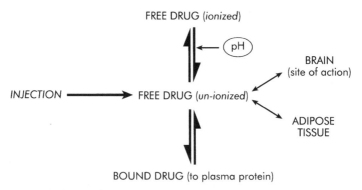

Figure 4.5 The distribution of an intravenously injected drug.

the arterial system it will reach the brain but it will only start to have its effect once diffusion across the lipid membranes has occurred. The effect of sedation will normally commence in one arm–brain circulation time, approximately 25 seconds. The final plasma concentration of the sedation agent will depend on the total dose of drug, the rate of the injection, the cardiac output and the circulating blood volume. The greater the dose of drug injected and the faster the rate of injection then the higher will be the plasma concentration. In contrast, the higher the cardiac output and higher the blood volume, the lower the plasma concentration.

Recovery from sedation occurs by two processes (Figure 4.6). The first is the redistribution of the sedation agent from the central nervous system into the body fat. The initial peak plasma concentration forces the sedation agent into tissues which are well perfused such as the brain, heart, liver and kidneys. With time an increasing amount of the sedation agent is taken into adipose tissue. Although solubility in fat is lower than in well-perfused tissues, the high mass of the body fat and the lipid solubility of sedation agents does promote redistribution to the fat stores. Ultimately the plasma concentration of drug falls and the blood–brain concentration gradient is reversed. This forces the sedation agent out of the brain and back into the blood stream. The second process involves the uptake and metabolism of the sedation agent in the liver and elimination via the kidneys. This results in the final reduction in plasma concentration leading to complete recovery of the patient.

The relative importance of redistribution and elimination depends on the individual sedation agent but in general, redistribution is responsible for the initial recovery from sedation (the alpha half-life), followed by elimination of the remaining drug (the beta half-life). Virtually all intravenous agents have two half-lives. Only those with very rapid metabolism do not demonstrate a biphasic curve. In considering different drugs, however, it is the elimination half-life which can be used to compare the pharmacokinetic effects of different sedation agents.

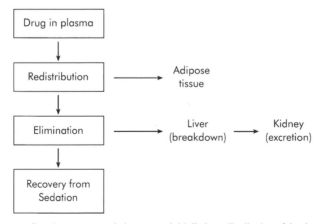

Figure 4.6 Recovery from intravenous sedation occurs initially by redistribution of the drug into adipose tissue followed by elimination of the drug by the liver and kidney.

Types of sedatives

The benzodiazepines

It was not until the 1960s that agents were developed specifically for conscious sedation. At this time a group of tranquillizing drugs known as the 'benzodiaze-pines' were discovered in Switzerland by researchers at Hoffman-La Roche. Since then the benzodiazepines have become the mainstay of modern sedation practice. They have been researched extensively and their mode of action is probably better understood than most other drugs.

In order to understand the mechanism of action of the benzodiazepines it is necessary to appreciate the normal passage of information through sensory neurones to the central nervous system. A system made up of 'GABA' (gamma-aminobutyric acid) receptors is responsible for filtering or damping down sensory input to the brain. GABA is an inhibitory chemical which is released from sensory nerve endings as electrical nerve stimuli pass from neurone to neurone over synapses. Once released, GABA attaches itself to receptors on the cell membrane of the post-synaptic neurone. The post-synaptic membrane becomes more permeable to chloride ions which has the effect of stabilizing the neurone and increasing the threshold for firing (Figure 4.7). During this refractory period no further electrical stimuli can be transmitted across the synapse. In this way the number of sensory messages which travel the whole distance of the neurones from their origin to the areas of the brain where they are perceived are reduced or filtered. For every stimulus to the senses (touch, taste, smell, hearing, sight, pain), very many more electrical stimuli are initiated than are necessary for the subject to perceive the stimulus and react to it.

Benzodiazepines act throughout the central nervous system via the GABA network. Specific benzodiazepine receptors are located close to GABA re-ceptors on neuronal membranes within the brain and spinal cord. All benzo-diazepines (which, like all sedatives, are central nervous system depressants) have a similar shape, with a ring structure on the same position of the dia-zepine part of each molecule (Figure 4.8). It is this common core shape which

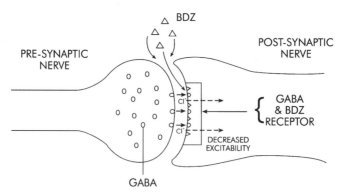

Figure 4.7 Mechanism of action of gamma-aminobutyric acid (GABA). GABA is released from the pre-synaptic sensory nerve ending, passes across the synapse and attaches to a GABA receptor on the post-synaptic neurone. This increases the permeability of the post-synaptic neurone to chloride ions, reducing the excitability of the nerve and preventing the passage of sensory stimuli. Benzodiazepine (BDZ) receptors are located close to the GABA receptor complex and BDZs produce a similar inhibitory effect on neural transmission.

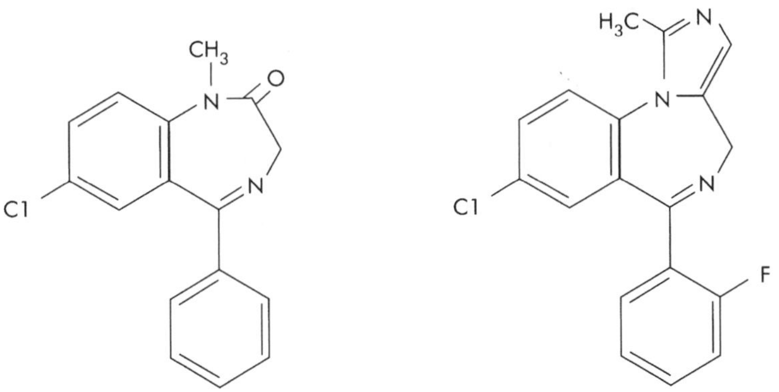

Figure 4.8 Chemical structure of the benzodiazepines, diazepam and midazolam. Both have a benzene ring structure attached to the diazepine part of the molecule.

enables them to attach to the benzodiazepine receptors. The effect of having a benzodiazepine in place on a receptor is to prolong the time it takes for re-polarization after a neurone has been depolarized by an electrical impulse. This further reduces the number of stimuli reaching the higher centres and produces pharmacological sedation, anxiolysis, amnesia, muscle relaxation and anticonvulsant effects. Benzodiazepines act essentially by mimicking the normal physiological filter system of the body and they may do so positively or negatively.

There is a range of benzodiazepines which varies from those having the desired effects (agonists) to those having the entirely opposite effect (inverse agonists). In the centre of the spectrum is a group of drugs which has an affinity for the benzodiazepine receptor but which is, to all intents and purposes, pharmacologically inactive (antagonists). Between the midpoint and the extremes are drugs which exhibit some limited effect but one which is less profound than would be anticipated (the partial agonists/partial inverse agonists). Because the drugs are all chemically similar, it is often only by animal testing that the real effects of an experimental benzodiazepine can be established.

The agonist benzodiazepines induce a state of conscious sedation with acute detachment for 20–30 minutes and a state of relaxation for a further hour or so. They also produce anterograde amnesia, muscle relaxation and have an anticonvulsant action. There is minimal cardiovascular and respiratory depression when intravenous benzodiazepines are titrated slowly to a defined end point of conscious sedation in healthy patients (titration refers to the process of delivering small increments of a sedative whilst observing the clinical response until it is deemed adequate). Benzodiazepines do not produce any clinically useful analgesia, although the sedation itself may alter the patient's response to pain (not always beneficially!).

Although the intravenous benzodiazepines are generally very safe sedation agents they do have some disadvantages. The most significant side effect is respiratory depression. Some degree of respiratory depression occurs in all patients sedated with the benzodiazepines but this usually only becomes clinically significant in patients with impaired respiratory function or in those who have taken other CNS depressants. A patient with pre-existing respiratory disease will already have a degree of respiratory compromise. They will be especially at risk from the respiratory depressant effects of the benzodiazepines. Similarly there is a synergistic relationship between the benzodiazepines and certain other CNS depressants, such as the opiates or alcohol. In a synergistic relationship the effect of two drugs is greater than the sum total of the individual drugs and this is particularly noticeable with the opiates when required doses may be 25% or less than if a single drug had been administered. The risk, therefore, of overdose in combined drug techniques is significantly higher than when a single agent is used and this was the rationale behind the restrictions in the Poswillo definition of simple sedation (see Chapter 1).

Excessively rapid intravenous injection of the benzodiazepines can cause significant respiratory depression which may result in apnoea. This can be avoided by slow incremental injection of the drug. If apnoea does occur then assisted ventilation will be required. It is also thought that the laryngeal reflexes may be momentarily obtunded immediately following injection of a benzodiazepine. Although this state is short-lived, the dental surgeon should always ensure that the patient's airway is well protected when performing dental treatment on sedated patients. Because of the risk of apnoea, the Royal College of Surgeons Report (1993) suggested the use of supplemental oxygen in all patients. At the current time this is not a universally accepted practice and it is questionable as to whether it is really indicated in fit, young healthy patients. There is little doubt, however, that supplemental oxygen does result in the maintenance of better oxygen saturation and it should, therefore, be considered particularly in older or medically compromised patients.

The benzodiazepines also produce minor cardiovascular side effects in healthy patients. They cause a reduction in vascular resistance which would normally result in a fall in blood pressure. This is compensated by an increase in heart rate and the cardiac output so that the blood pressure is minimally unaffected.

Elderly patients are particularly susceptible to the effects of the benzodiazepines. It is relatively easy to overdose an older patient and cause significant respiratory depression. Intravenous benzodiazepines should be administered slowly and in very small increments to the elderly. The total dose required to produce sedation will be much smaller than in a younger adult of the equivalent weight. Intravenous benzodiazepines should be avoided in children in dental practice. Children react unpredictably to intravenous benzodiazepines and can easily become over-sedated. Occasionally they become extremely distraught and this may be more common in the teenage years. Extreme care needs to be undertaken with such patients as the temptation to keep adding further increments can easily result in an unconscious patient.

Patients who are already taking oral benzodiazepines for anxiolysis or insomnia may be tolerant to the effect of intravenous benzodiazepines. Those who have become dependent on long-term benzodiazepine therapy may also have their dependence reactivated by acute intravenous administration. There have also been reported incidents of sexual fantasy occurring under intravenous benzodiazepine sedation but this only seems to occur when higher than recommended doses of the drug are administered. Providing recommended protocols are followed, this should not be a problem with any of the agents in common usage.

Diazepam   Diazepam was the first benzodiazepine to be used in intravenous sedation practice. It is almost insoluble in water and so it is either dissolved in the organic solvent, propylene glycol (Valium®), or it is emulsified into a suspension in soya bean oil (Diazemuls®). The organic solvent formulation caused a high incidence of vein damage, ranging from pain to frank thrombophlebitis and even skin ulceration, so this preparation is no longer used. Diazemuls is a non-irritant preparation which overcomes the problem of venous damage. Diazepam is metabolized in the liver and eliminated via the kidneys. It has a long elimination half-life of 43 hours (±13 hours) although its $t_{1/2}\alpha$ is in the region of 40 minutes. An active metabolite, n-desmethyldiazepam, is produced which can cause rebound sedation up to 72 hours after the initial administration of diazepam. Diazemuls is presented in a 2-ml ampoule in a concentration of 5 mg/ml for intravenous injection. It is a reliable hypnosedative which should be given slowly, titrating the dose against the response obtained. The standard dose lies in the range 0.1–0.2 mg/kg. Unfortunately the long recovery period and possibility of rebound sedation mean that diazepam in any form is not the ideal drug for sedation for short dental procedures and its use has largely been superseded by the more modern and more rapidly metabolized midazolam.

Midazolam   Midazolam was introduced into clinical practice in 1983 although it had been synthesized several years previously. It is currently the agent of choice for intravenous sedation in dentistry although there are newer agents on the horizon. It is a benzodiazepine which is water soluble with a pH of less than 4.0 and which is non-irritant to veins. Once injected into the blood stream, at physiological pH, it becomes lipid soluble and is readily able to penetrate the blood–brain barrier. It has an elimination half-life $(t_{1/2}\beta)$ of 1.9 hours (±0.9 hours) so that complete recovery is quicker than that with diazepam. Midazolam is more rapidly acting, at least two and a half times as potent and has more predictable amnesic properties than diazepam. It is rapidly metabolized in the liver but there is also some extra-hepatic metabolism in the bowel. Midazolam produces an active metabolite called alpha-hydroxymidazolam. This has a short half-life of 1.25 hours (±0.25 hours) which is less than that of the parent compound and thus does not produce true rebound sedation. It does, however, explain the clinically observable phenomenon of a slower initial recovery from midazolam sedation than would be expected on the basis of the pharmacokinetics of the drug without reference to its active metabolite.

Midazolam is presented in two forms: at a concentration of 5 mg/ml in a 2-ml ampoule or at a concentration of 2 mg/ml in a 5-ml ampoule. Both presentations contain the same quantity of midazolam but the 5 ml (2 mg/ml) presentation, being less concentrated, is easier to titrate and is more acceptable for use in dental practice. The dose of midazolam is titrated according to the patient's response but most patients require a dose usually in the range of 0.06–0.1 mg/kg.

Flumazenil   The discovery of the benzodiazepine antagonist, flumazenil, in 1978, was a major advance in the practice of intravenous sedation. This is the first drug to effectively and completely reverse the effects of almost all benzodiazepines. Flumazenil is a true benzodiazepine but it has virtually no intrinsic therapeutic activity (the administration of huge doses of flumazenil may result in very slight epileptiform activity). It shares the same basic chemical

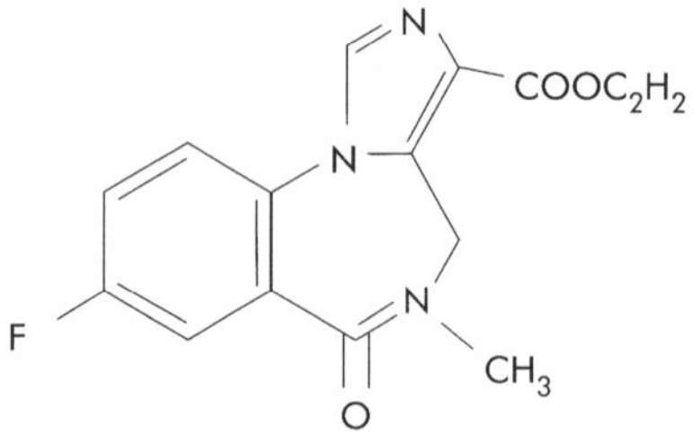

Flumazenil

Figure 4.9 Chemical structure of flumazenil, the benzodiazepine antagonist. The molecule has no benzene ring attached to the diazepine group.

form as other benzodiazepines but it lacks the ring structure attached to the diazepine part of the molecule (Figure 4.9). It is this slight alteration in structure which probably prevents flumazenil from having any genuine therapeutic activity. Flumazenil has a greater affinity for the benzodiazepine receptor than virtually all the known active drugs and it is therefore an effective antagonist. It will reverse the sedative, cardiovascular and respiratory depressant effects of both diazepam and midazolam, in fact the vast majority of all commercially available benzodiazepines.

Flumazenil is presented in 5-ml ampoules containing 100 μg/ml for intravenous injection. It is administered by giving 200 μg and then waiting for 1 minute. A further 100 μg is then given every minute until the patient appears fully recovered. In an acute emergency there is no reason why a higher initial dose of up to 500 μg should not be given immediately as a bolus. Flumazenil is currently only recommended for use in an emergency situation and not as a means of hastening recovery. If flumazenil were used for routine reversal there is a theoretical risk that the benzodiazepine sedation may recur once the effect of the flumazenil had worn off. This is because flumazenil has a shorter elimination half-life (about 50 minutes) than the active benzodiazepines. For healthy patients this is a theoretical concept with little relevance to clinical practice and the greatest objections to using flumazenil routinely are its cost and the rather sudden and unpleasant 'wakening' which it produces.

Other intravenous sedation agents
Although the benzodiazepines are the mainstay of modern sedation practice they do not fulfil all the requirements of the ideal sedation drug. The main problem is the relatively long period of recovery that is required before a patient can be discharged home and return to normal daily activities. Pharmaceutical companies are unlikely to invent the ideal sedation agent, i.e. one which will meet the criteria specified at the beginning of this chapter due, at least in part, to the high cost of developing any new drug. To date there is only one drug which appears to have serious potential as the sedation agent of the future.

Propofol is a short-acting, intravenous general anaesthetic agent, which has found widespread acceptability especially as an induction agent for day-case general anaesthesia. It is presented as an aqueous white emulsion at a concentration of 10 mg/ml in 20-ml ampoules (Figure 4.10). It has the advantage of undergoing rapid elimination and recovery with a distribution half-life of 2–4 minutes and an elimination half-life of 30–40 minutes. For maintenance of general anaesthesia, propofol is administered as a continuous infusion. Following completion of the operative procedure, the infusion is stopped and the patient regains consciousness within a few minutes.

Clinical trials using propofol in differing ways for dental sedation have been promising. Incremental doses of propofol are administered initially until a satisfactory level of sedation is achieved, usually at a total dose of around 0.5 mg/kg. The desired level of sedation is maintained by delivering a continuous infusion of around 1.5–4.5 mg/kg/hr. The infusion rate can be adjusted to vary the level of sedation as required. Once treatment is complete the infusion is switched off and the patient will normally be fully recovered and fit to be discharged home within 10–15 minutes. Clinical trials using propofol administered through a patient-controlled infusion pump (similar to those used for postoperative analgesia) have also been very promising and these are detailed in Chapter 5.

In many ways, propofol approaches the requirements of an ideal sedation agent. However, it does have a number of disadvantages. The margin of safety between sedation and anaesthesia is far narrower than that of the benzodiazepines. Special equipment is also needed as the administration of propofol is by continuous infusion, requiring the use of a special infusion pump. Injection of propofol can also be painful and it should preferably be delivered into larger veins or following pre-injection with a local anaesthetic. The use of propofol for dental sedation is essentially still at the experimental stage and as such it can only be currently recommended for use in a hospital environment.

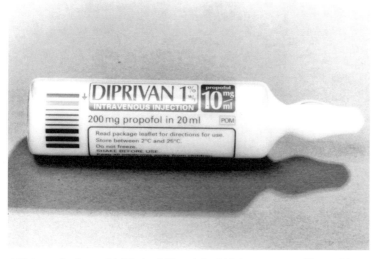

Figure 4.10 Ampoule of propofol (Diprivan) 10 mg/ml, which is an aqueous white emulsion.

References and further reading

Cook, P.J., Flanagan, R. and James, I.M. (1984). Diazepam tolerance: effect of age, regular sedation and alcohol. *British Medical Journal*, **289**, 351.

Greenblatt, D.J., Shader, R.I. and Abernethy, D.R. (1993). Current status of the benzodiazepines. *New England Journal of Medicine*, **309**, 354.

Mackenzie, N. and Grant, I.S. (1987). Propofol for intravenous sedation. *Anaesthesia*, **42**, 3–6.

Richards, A., Griffiths, M. and Scully, C. (1993). Wide variation in patient response to midazolam sedation for out-patient oral surgery. *Oral Surgery, Oral Medicine and Oral Pathology*, **76**, 408–411.

Rosenbaum, N.R. (1988). Flumazenil as an antagonist to midazolam in intravenous sedation for dental procedures. *European Journal of Anaesthesiology*, Suppl. 2, 183–190.

5

Inhalational sedation: principles and practice

Introduction

Inhalational sedation is the safest form of sedation, due principally to the nature of nitrous oxide which is almost universally used in this technique. The term 'inhalational sedation' describes the induction of a state of conscious sedation by administering subanaesthetic concentrations of gaseous anaesthetic agents. Its most common application is in children's dentistry, where it has been used successfully for many decades but its use in adult dentistry is certainly not rare. The favourable pharmacological properties of nitrous oxide make this the agent of choice for most inhalational sedation techniques. Ever since its discovery, nitrous oxide has been the basic constituent of gaseous general anaesthesia although it was not until the 1960s that it was more widely exploited for use in inhalational sedation although, as mentioned previously, it was used in the Scandinavian countries from the time of the First World War. In the early 1960s, however, Harold Langa in the United States introduced the concept of 'relative analgesia', a specific type of inhalational sedation which uses variable mixtures of nitrous oxide and oxygen to induce a state of psychopharmacological sedation. Relative analgesia comes under the umbrella of the first stage of anaesthesia.

The staging of inhalational anaesthesia dates back to the days when the standard agent was ether. Di-ethyl ether was first synthesized in 1540 and was used as an anaesthetic agent from 1840. Its high blood–gas partition coefficient (circa 13) resulted in prolonged induction of anaesthesia often accompanied by much involuntary struggling by the patient. The stages of anaesthesia were described by Guedel and were based on induction of anaesthesia using ether; although found in all standard textbooks of anaesthesia, they are no longer recognizable with today's modern, rapidly effective agents.

Langa, however, developed the concept of 'planes of analgesia' within Stage 1 of anaesthesia (see below) and relative analgesia has now become the standard technique for inhalational sedation in dentistry. Other methods of inhalational sedation do exist, such as the use of fixed concentrations of nitrous oxide and oxygen (entonox), but these are not commonly used in dentistry.

Relative analgesia sedation

The aims of relative analgesia sedation are to alleviate fear by producing anxiolysis, to reduce pain by inducing analgesia and to improve patient co-operation so that dental treatment can be performed. The term 'relative analgesia' embodies a triad of three elements:

1. The administration of low to moderate titrated concentrations of nitrous oxide in oxygen to patients who remain conscious.
2. The use of a machine which is designed specifically for relative analgesia. It must have a number of safety features, including the ability to deliver a minimum of 30% oxygen and a fail-safe device that cuts off the delivery of nitrous oxide if the oxygen supply fails.
3. The use of semi-hypnotic suggestion to reassure and encourage the patient throughout the period of sedation and treatment.

The success of sedation produced with relative analgesia relies on a balanced combination of pharmacology and behavioural management. Nitrous oxide will produce a degree of pharmacological sedation on its own but this is unpredictable and needs to be supplemented and reinforced with psychological reassurance. The pharmacological properties of nitrous oxide produce physiological changes which enhance the patient's susceptibility to suggestion. The use of semi-hypnotic suggestion to positively reinforce feelings of relaxation and well-being will increase the extent of the anxiolysis and co-operation. In contrast to intravenous sedation which produces pharmacological sedation regardless of any element of suggestion, relative analgesia induces a state of psychopharmacological sedation.

Planes of analgesia

The clinical effects of sedation with nitrous oxide can be divided into three broad categories. These form part of the 'stages of anaesthesia' which were originally described by Guedel (Figure 5.1). The first stage of anaesthesia, the analgesic stage, is subdivided into three 'planes of analgesia':

Plane I   Moderate sedation and analgesia, obtained with concentrations of 5–25% nitrous oxide.
Plane II   Dissociation sedation and analgesia, occurring at concentrations of 20–55% nitrous oxide.
Plane III Total analgesia, obtained with concentrations of nitrous oxide usually well above 50%.

In general terms, most clinically useful sedation is produced in Plane I and sometimes in Plane II, although some patients find the dissociation effects a little disorientating. It is these planes which are encompassed by the definition of relative analgesia. Plane III is a transition zone between the state of conscious sedation and true general anaesthesia and thus it is termed 'total analgesia' rather than 'relative analgesia'. There is considerable overlap between the planes and a large variation in susceptibility of individual patients to the effects of nitrous oxide. Whilst one person may be adequately sedated with 10% nitrous oxide, another individual may require in excess of 50% nitrous oxide to achieve the same degree of sedation.

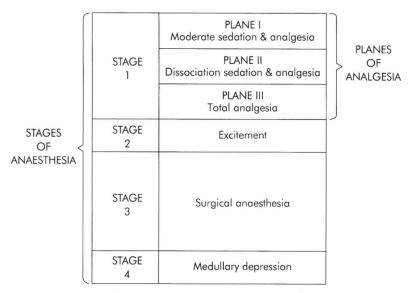

Figure 5.1 Guedel's stages of anaesthesia. Stage 1 is subdivided into three planes of analgesia.

Each plane of analgesia is accompanied by specific clinical signs (Figure 5.2). At the onset of Plane I (N_2O concentrations of 5–25%), the patient will be relaxed and feel a general sense of well-being. There may well be paraesthesia of the extremities—a tingling feeling, particularly the fingers, toes and cheeks; a feeling of suffusing warmth is also common. The patient will be awake and will respond readily to questioning. There will be a slight reduction

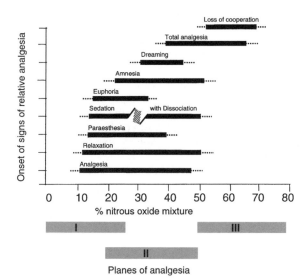

Figure 5.2 Clinical effects seen during different planes of analgesia. These signs are variable and some are more predictable than others.

in spontaneous movements and a decreased reaction to painful stimuli. The pulse, blood pressure, respiration rate, reflexes and pupil reactions will all be normal.

As the nitrous oxide concentration is increased into the 20–55% range there will be a gradual transition from Plane I into Plane II. The patient will become very relaxed and sleepy and may feel detached from the environment. Their senses will be altered and they may experience dreaming. They will have widespread paraesthesia, moderate analgesia and a reduction in the gag reflex. Although the patient will be awake there will be a delayed response to questioning. Vital signs and the laryngeal reflexes should be unaffected.

When the nitrous oxide concentration goes above 50% there will be a transition into Plane III. The patient will become very sleepy and will have a glazed appearance. There will be complete analgesia and the patient may complain of nausea and dizziness and may actually vomit. Ultimately the patient will become unresponsive to questioning, will lose consciousness and may enter Stage 2 of general anaesthesia. This may be accompanied by restlessness and/or struggling. If this occurs the nitrous oxide level should be reduced.

There is usually a gradual transition between planes and not all patients show all the clinical signs. However, the planes of analgesia are a useful guide of what to expect when sedating a patient with nitrous oxide. Specific signs such as nausea, dizziness and a glazed appearance provide a warning that the level of sedation is too high and the percentage of nitrous oxide should be reduced. However, there is considerable variation in individual response and it should be remembered at all times that the success of the technique is probably more dependent on the operator's ability to infuse hypnotic suggestion than it is to the effect of nitrous oxide!

Indications and contra-indications for relative analgesia

Relative analgesia is primarily indicated for the management of dental anxiety, especially in children. It should be viewed as part of an overall behaviour management strategy. Many children are apprehensive about receiving routine operative dentistry and require some extra support to help them to accept treatment. It is important to determine whether anxiety stems from a lack of understanding (in very young children) or a fear of the unknown. It might also have arisen as a result of a traumatic past experience or from adverse parental conditioning. One particular feature of this is the experience of 'having the gas' at the dentists and children who have heard vivid accounts of bad experiences of this nature from their parents are not likely to appreciate inhalational sedation unless it is very carefully introduced.

Children must be able to understand the purpose and mechanisms (in appropriate terminology) of inhalation sedation and so the minimum age for treating children under relative analgesia is approximately 3 years. This is usually the lowest age at which the child has an appropriate degree of understanding to enable sufficient co-operation for treatment under relative analgesia. Most children of 3 years and older will be amenable to receiving routine restorative dentistry and simple extraction of deciduous teeth under relative analgesia. Older children scheduled for orthodontic extractions may also benefit from relative analgesia. Such children may not be particularly frightened of routine treatment but multiple extractions of permanent teeth or surgical procedures, such as the exposure of canines, can be somewhat traumatic. Sedation can help to make the procedure more acceptable and the time pass more quickly.

Another key indication for relative analgesia is the treatment of adults who have a general (as opposed to dental) phobia of needles or injections. Such individuals find it impossible to accept venepuncture and venous cannulation. They can benefit considerably from relative analgesia, either as the sole form of sedation or in combination with intravenous sedation. In many cases the level of sedation and analgesia achieved with relative analgesia is sufficient for the patient to receive a local anaesthetic injection into the mucosa with minimal discomfort and simple operative dentistry can then be performed. However, for patients with a severe anxiety or phobia of dentistry, it may be necessary to supplement relative analgesia with an intravenous technique. In these individuals the relative analgesia is used to induce a level of sedation sufficient to enable venous cannulation to be performed. Once the cannula is successfully located, the intravenous sedative can be administered and the delivery of nitrous oxide terminated.

Relative analgesia is also used for a number of special categories of patients, who are at risk from the respiratory depressive effects of intravenous agents. These include, for example, patients with sickle cell anaemia or severe asthma, who benefit from the guaranteed level of oxygenation (at least 30% and usually significantly more) used in relative analgesia. For the few patients with a proven allergy to intravenous sedatives, the only alternative sedation technique may be relative analgesia. Pregnant women in the second or third trimester may also find relative analgesia useful, especially if intravenous sedation is contra-indicated.

Many of the contra-indications to inhalational sedation are relative or temporary. Nitrous oxide is administered via a nose mask or nasal cannula and thus successful inhalation requires a patent nasal airway. Upper respiratory tract infections, large tonsils or adenoids, or serious respiratory disease contra-indicate the use of relative analgesia. As mentioned, very young children do not usually have enough understanding to be able to interact and co-operate for successful relative analgesia. Older children who have had an inhalational anaesthetic in earlier years may develop a fear of the anaesthetic mask. The nose mask used in relative analgesia appears very similar to an anaesthetic mask to the wary child and as such cannot be used. Patients with moderate to severe learning difficulties or those who have severe psychiatric disorders are also not suitable for relative analgesia. Pregnant women in the first trimester of pregnancy should not be given nitrous oxide because of the potential teratogenic effect on the foetus. Finally, the position of the nose mask makes operative dentistry on the labial aspect of the upper maxilla difficult; for example it would be difficult to perform an apicectomy on an upper incisor using relative analgesia unless the nasal cannula is used.

Very few of the indications and contra-indications for relative analgesia are absolute. In many cases it is necessary to balance the risk of giving the patient sedation against the risk of administering general anaesthesia, which is often the only option for many severely anxious dental patients. Each patient should be individually assessed and only those who fit the above selection criteria and who meet the general standards discussed in Chapter 3 should be treated in dental practice. There may be others, however, who can be referred for treatment under relative analgesia in a hospital setting where any complications can be dealt with more easily.

Patient preparation for relative analgesia

Assessment and treatment planning for patients for relative analgesia should follow the format described earlier (see Chapter 3). The only difference is that most patients presenting for relative analgesia are children. It is undoubtedly preferable to involve both the child and the parent in the assessment appointment. With children it can be difficult to determine whether the patient actually needs sedation or not. Children can be very unpredictable and those who initially appear calm and relaxed at examination can suddenly become unco-operative once an attempt is made to administer local anaesthesia. Children are inherently apprehensive about having operative dental treatment, largely because of fear of the unknown. Relative analgesia should be seen as a part of an overall behaviour management strategy and the aim of the assessment appointment should be to select those who really do need some form of extra support to help them through treatment.

The type and extent of dental treatment needed should be taken into account when considering sedation. Although most routine operative dentistry can be performed under relative analgesia, the nature of the treatment must be matched against the age of the patient and their predicted level of co-operation. One or two extractions in a 4 year old could, quite reasonably, be performed under relative analgesia. However, if the same patient required the extraction of multiple grossly carious teeth it might be kinder to refer the patient for a short general anaesthetic.

Similarly, a 13 year old could willingly accept the extraction of four pre-molars under relative analgesia but if the exposure of a deeply buried canine is required then general anaesthesia may be preferable.

Assessment of the medical status of a patient scheduled for relative analgesia is identical to that described in Chapter 3. Particular attention should be paid to respiratory disease as this can affect ventilation and gas exchange. The child should be examined to check patency of the nasal air passages. A baseline pulse and respiration rate should be recorded but, for healthy children, it is unnecessary to take the weight and blood pressure. A full explanation of the procedure should be given to both the child and the parent. The child should be told that they will be given some 'happy air' or 'magic wind' to breath which will make them feel 'warm', 'tingly' and 'sleepy'. Once they feel comfortable then their tooth will be 'wiggled out' or 'mended'. The truth should always be told although the use of good semantics is extremely important. The child should be reassured that they will be able to talk to the dentist while they are sedated and that they can reduce or increase the level of sedation by breathing through their mouth or nose respectively. Clearly the level of explanation should be individually pitched according to the age and level of understanding of the child. The parent, guardian or patient (if over the age of 16 years) should be asked to sign a written consent to both the sedation and dental treatment.

Full verbal and written instructions about pre- and postoperative care should be given to the parent or to the patient (if appropriate). Patients scheduled for relative analgesia should be starved for 2 hours prior to the appointment and children must be accompanied by a responsible escort. Adults who are undergoing relative analgesia, as the sole method of sedation, do not need to be accompanied. Once they are deemed fit for discharge adults can go home alone, although it is inadvisable for them to drive.

Equipment for relative analgesia

Machines have been designed specifically for use in relative analgesia. The Quantiflex MDM® is the standard machine used in the United Kingdom (Figure 5.3). It allows a variable percentage of nitrous oxide and oxygen to be delivered to the patient via a nose mask. The gas flow is continuous but the rate can be individually adjusted to match the patient's minute volume.

The Quantiflex MDM® is a free-standing machine which carries its own gas supply—two cylinders of nitrous oxide and two cylinders of oxygen. One cylinder of each gas is in active use and the second cylinder is a reserve supply which must always be kept full and should be labelled accordingly. The active cylinders are attached to the machine via a specific pin-index connection which prevents attachment of the wrong gas cylinders. Gas leaving the cylinders goes through a pressure reducing valve before passing into a flow control head (Figure 5.4). The flow rate of each gas can be visualized in two flowmeters on the control head, each calibrated in increments up to 10 litres per minute. The nitrous oxide and oxygen are mixed in the flow control head. A flow control knob regulates the rate at which the gas mixture is delivered to the patient and a mixture control dial determines the relative percentage of nitrous oxide and oxygen being delivered to the patient. The mixture control dial actually indicates the percentage of oxygen being administered and is

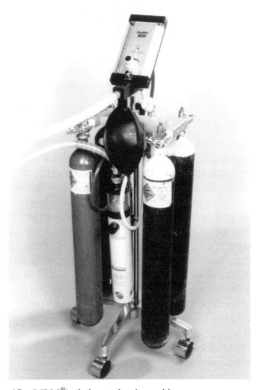

Figure 5.3 The Quantiflex MDM® relative analgesia machine.

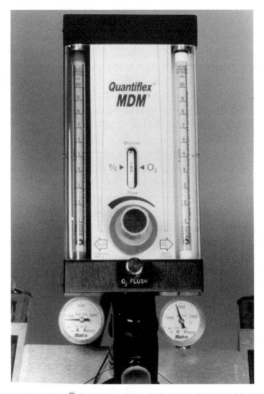

Figure 5.4 The Quantiflex MDM® flow control head, showing nitrous oxide and oxygen flowmeters, mixture control dial, flow control knob and oxygen flush button. Below the control head are the pressure gauges for the nitrous oxide (left) and oxygen (right) cylinders.

marked in 10% increments, from 100% to 30%. As the oxygen concentration is changed the balance of the gas mixture is automatically made to 100% with nitrous oxide. For example, if the percentage of oxygen is 70% the percentage of nitrous oxide will automatically be set by the machine at 30%. The control head also contains an air entrainment valve which opens automatically to let air in if there is any negative pressure in the breathing circuit. So if the gas flow rate is inadvertently set too low for a particular patient the air entrainment valve will open so that the patient can breath room air in addition to the delivered gas volume.

After leaving the flow control head the gas mixture enters a reservoir bag (Figure 5.5) which has three main purposes. First, it allows the flow rate to be accurately adjusted to match the patient's individual minute volume. If the bag empties whilst the patient breaths then the flow rate is set too low for that patient's minute volume. In contrast, if the bag is continuously over-inflated and the escape valve leaking, then the flow rate is set too high. Ideally the reservoir bag should stay about three-quarters full, deflating slightly as the patient inspires and refilling as the patient expires.

The second use of the reservoir bag is as an adjunct to clinical monitoring. Regular observation of movement of the bag during treatment allows the dental

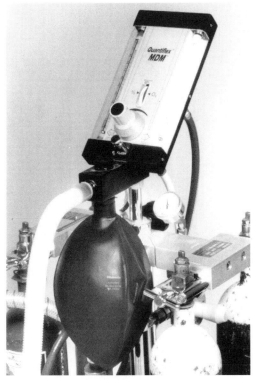

Figure 5.5 The reservoir bag is sited just below the flow control head. It is used to monitor the patient's breathing and to adjust the gas flow rate.

surgeon to monitor the respiration rate and depth. It is often easier to monitor respiration by observing the reservoir bag than by looking for chest movement, especially if the chest is covered by a protective bib.

The final use of the reservoir bag is for manual positive pressure ventilation in the event of an emergency.

The gas mixture is administered to the patient via a gas delivery hose attached to the input port of a suitable nasal mask. There are various sizes of rubber nose masks available and it is important to select one which provides the best seal with the patient's face (Figure 5.6). A poorly fitting mask will allow gas to escape and this not only decreases the efficiency of the sedation but also leads to pollution of the dental surgery. The patient inhales fresh gas from the mask and then exhales waste gas back into the mask. Exhaled gas passes via the output port in the mask into a scavenging hose. A one-way valve in the scavenging hose prevents waste gas from being re-inhaled. The exhaled gas either moves passively down the expiratory hose or is actively removed by a customized scavenging system.

The Quantiflex MDM machine has two specific features which are designed to maximize the safety of relative analgesia. First, the machine is set so that the minimum oxygen delivery is 30% of total gas volume, regardless of the total volume of gases flowing. The mixture control dial cannot be adjusted to

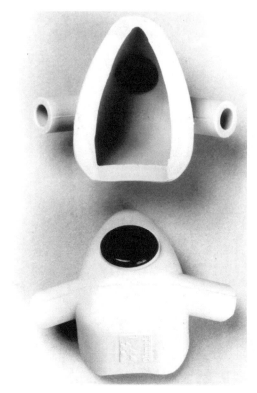

Figure 5.6 Nose mask used for relative analgesia.

percentages lower than 30% oxygen so the patient will always receive a gas mixture with a higher percentage of oxygen than is present in normal room air (> 21%). Consequently, it is impossible to deliver more than 70% nitrous oxide to the patient, so the chances of inducing full anaesthesia are remote.

The second safety feature is an automatic cut-out of all gas delivery if the oxygen supply fails and the oxygen delivery falls below 30%. This would only occur if the oxygen cylinder ran out of gas or if there was blockage or leakage in the high pressure system. This feature also ensures that 100% nitrous oxide can never be delivered to the patient.

Before proceeding to administer inhalational sedation it is essential that a thorough pre-operative check of all the equipment is made. This needs to be systematically and routinely completed.

Equipment checks
The relative analgesia machine and associated apparatus should always be thoroughly checked before use. Each oxygen cylinder must be separately switched on and the pressure dial checked. One cylinder at least should be completely full and any cylinders showing low readings should be changed. The flow rate should be turned on to maximum and the dial rechecked to ensure that there is no decrease in pressure. If such a decrease occurs it would indicate that either the quantity of gas in the cylinder is low or there is an obstruction in the

high pressure part of the system. The 'full' cylinder should then be switched off and labelled as full. Cylinders of nitrous oxide need to be weighed to confirm the quantity of gas. Nitrous oxide is stored as a liquid under pressure and the pressure dial will not accurately indicate the amount of liquid in the cylinder. The ability to deliver a sufficient flow of gas should also be tested.

A check should be made for leaks in the system by occluding the nose mask with one hand, allowing the reservoir bag to fill up and then squeezing it hard. The bag should not deflate unless gas is forced through the nose mask past the occluding hand. Any other deflation of the bag indicates a leakage. Leakages at the cylinder head indicate the need to replace the rubber washer known as the Bodok seal.

The effectiveness of the safety cut-out should then be tested by switching on both oxygen and nitrous oxide, setting the mixture control dial to 50% oxygen/50% nitrous oxide and the flow rate to 8 litres/minute. When the oxygen cylinder is turned off, the nitrous oxide should automatically cut-out within a few seconds.

The oxygen flush button should be tested, the gas hoses inspected and the one-way valve in the expiratory limb of the breathing system should be in place. If an active scavenging system is available the expiratory hose should be connected.

Finally the correct cylinders should be switched on and their valves opened fully. The equipment is now ready to be used. A checklist of the above procedures is shown in Figure 5.7.

SAFETY CHECKLIST FOR RELATIVE ANALGESIA

- Check the oxygen cylinders by reading their pressure gauges. Weigh the nitrous oxide cylinders.

- Change any cylinder that is approaching empty.

- Open the gas cylinder valves fully and check there is no leaking.

- Press the emergency oxygen flow button, whilst observing the oxygen pressure meter, which

- Open the nitrous oxide and oxygen valves to at least 5 litres per minutes.

- Whilst the gases are flowing block the mask or tubing to inflate the reservoir bag. Squeeze the bag to make sure it can generate a positive pressure against the blocked tubing.

- Whilst the gases are flowing, turn off the oxygen cylinder and check that the safety mechanism cuts off the nitrous oxide.

- Turn off all the gases on the machine valves and at the cylinders if they are not being used in the near future.

Figure 5.7 A safety checklist to ensure correct operation of the machinery. It can also be helpful to have a separate list to check the patient prior to giving relative analgesia or intravenous sedation, see Chapter 6.

Relative analgesia technique

All the equipment should be placed unobtrusively so that the patient is not unduly frightened when they come into the room. The patient should be brought into the surgery and settled in the dental chair. The procedure for relative analgesia is explained and the patient is told about the positive feelings they will have during sedation (Figure 5.8). They should be reassured that they will be able to talk to the dentist during treatment and that the level of sedation can be reduced simply by mouth breathing. It is better to recline the patient into a supine position before starting the sedation, as this makes the technique easier and minimizes the risk of fainting. Alternatively, the Trendelenburg position, where the patient is semi-supine with raised legs, may be more acceptable. Once the patient is comfortable an appropriately sized nose mask is selected and they are asked to place it on their nose. With children particularly, it is better if they perform this task themselves. If the size is correct then the mask is momentarily removed, connected to the gas hoses and repositioned on the patient's nose (Figure 5.9).

The flow rate required varies so in children the machine is set to deliver 100% oxygen at a flow rate of about 5 litres/minute. In adults an initial flow rate of about 8 litres/minute should be more than adequate. In either case it is usually better to start with slightly too much gas flowing than cause any feelings of suffocation from too little gas flowing. The patient is asked to try and keep their mouth closed and to breath slowly and regularly. They should be told that they are just receiving air and that they will not feel any sedation effects yet. A steady patter of conversation is required to encourage and reassure the patient. After a few minutes the flow rate is checked by asking the patient if they are getting the right amount of air, by looking at the patient to see if they are supplementing the flow by mouth breathing and by observing the inflation of the reservoir bag which should be comfortably full when the patient expires. The flow rate is adjusted (usually by reducing it) until a comfortable minute volume is achieved.

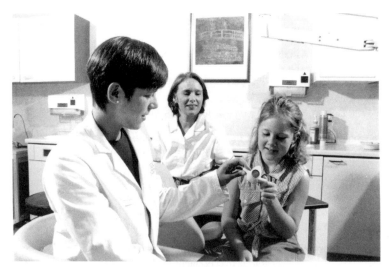

Figure 5.8 The procedure for relative analgesia is explained to the patient once they are settled in the dental chair.

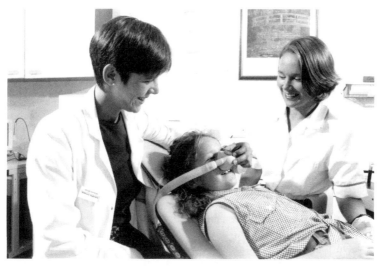

Figure 5.9 Once the gas hoses have been attached the nose mask is comfortably positioned on the patient's nose.

Assuming all is progressing uneventfully, the administration of nitrous oxide can then be slowly introduced. Ten percent nitrous oxide is added by turning the mixture control dial to 90% oxygen. Because of the design qualities of the Quantiflex MDM, this will not alter the overall gas volume. The patient should be told that they may begin to feel light headed with warm tingling of the hands and feet. They may also start to feel a little detached from their surroundings and experience changes in hearing and vision.

At this stage it is extremely important to reassure the patient by continuous conversation and encouragement, stressing that the feelings will be positive and pleasant. The flow is maintained for one full minute and then the concentration of nitrous oxide is increased by a further 10% increment, to 20% (80% oxygen) for a further full minute. Thereafter the level of nitrous oxide can be increased in 5% increments each minute, the dose being carefully titrated according to the patient's response.

It can be difficult to determine an appropriate end-point for nitrous oxide sedation. The objective signs of sedation which occur with intravenous techniques are not usually present with relative analgesia. An adequate level of sedation is achieved when there is general relaxation and the patient is less fidgety and less talkative, there is tingling or paraesthesia of the fingers, toes and possibly the lips and a slowed response to questioning.

Nitrous oxide concentrations between 20% and 50% commonly allow for a state of detached sedation and analgesia without any loss of consciousness or danger of obtunded laryngeal reflexes. At this level patients are aware of the operative procedure and co-operate without being fearful. With adults, they can simply be asked if they are feeling adequately relaxed and will usually respond appropriately; with children this is less reliable and so the dentist must attempt to assess the level of co-operation obtained.

If after a period of relaxation patients becomes restless and apprehensive, or if they start to complain of nausea or dizziness, this is usually an indication that the level of nitrous oxide is too high. The percentage of nitrous oxide should be reduced and the patient maintained at a more appropriate level until the operative procedure is complete. If at any time the patient becomes glazed and unresponsive to questioning, it is probably due to entering the early stages of anaesthesia and the immediate response should be to reduce the nitrous oxide level.

Once an appropriate level of sedation has been achieved local anaesthesia can be administered. The analgesic effect of nitrous oxide can make local anaesthetic injections almost painless, but it is still good practice to use a topical anaesthetic as well. Treatment can commence once the local anaesthetic has taken effect. Administration of nitrous oxide and oxygen should continue throughout the operative period and treatment should be accompanied by ongoing reassurance and encouragement. The degree of sedation may fall slightly during treatment as the gas mixture becomes diluted by mouth breathing. This can be rectified by ceasing dental treatment every few minutes and asking the patient to close their mouth and breath through their nose for a few minutes. On no account should a dental prop ever be used to keep the patient's mouth open during routine treatment. If a patient cannot maintain an open mouth then they are too deeply sedated.

It is essential to monitor the clinical status of the patient throughout the period of nitrous oxide sedation. Clinical monitoring of respiration rate and depth, pulse, colour, level of sedation and responsiveness are mandatory. However, in a healthy patient, it is not necessary to supplement clinical observation with electromechanical monitoring. Pulse oximetry and blood pressure measurement during relative analgesia are only indicated in the care of medically compromised patients, especially those with cardiac insufficiency. It is useful to have them available, however, in case of an untoward complication.

When dental treatment is complete the nitrous oxide flow is shut off and 100% oxygen is administered for two minutes. The aim of this is primarily to prevent diffusion hypoxia. Diffusion hypoxia is a condition which results from the rapid outflow of nitrous oxide across the alveolar membrane when the incoming gas flow is stopped. Even using relative analgesia this can dilute the percentage of alveolar oxygen available for uptake by up to 50% although the risk of severe, life-threatening diffusion hypoxia is very low. The administration of 100% oxygen counteracts the potential desaturation caused by diffusion hypoxia. It also speeds up recovery and helps to prevent surgery pollution by ensuring that exhaled air passes into the scavenging hose.

Finally the patient is asked to remove the face mask and is slowly brought back to the upright position. After a period of about 10–15 minutes the patient is usually fit to be discharged. The dental surgeon should check that the patient is coherent, steady on his/her feet and can walk unaided. Children should be discharged into the care of an adult, with verbal and written postoperative instructions (Figure 5.10). Adult patients can be allowed home unaccompanied once the dental surgeon has confirmed their fitness to be discharged.

Advantages and disadvantages of relative analgesia

In comparison with intravenous sedation, relative analgesia has a number of advantages. The technique is non-invasive and there is no requirement for

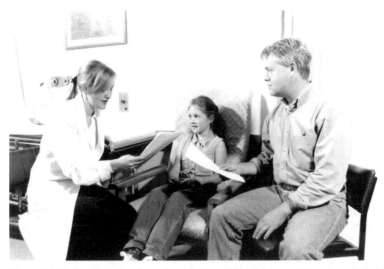

Figure 5.10 Before the patient is discharged after sedation it is essential to give verbal and written postoperative instructions to both the patient and escort.

venepuncture and cannulation. The drug is administered through the lungs and is relatively inert so that there are no metabolic demands and recovery is rapid. The favourable properties of nitrous oxide, in particular its low solubility, mean that the level of sedation can easily be altered or discontinued. There is little effect on the cardiovascular and respiratory systems and impairment of reflexes is minimal. Some analgesia is produced which can be helpful in obviating the discomfort of local anaesthetic injections.

Relative analgesia does also have some disadvantages. The main problem is that the drug has to be administered continuously via a mask which is close to the operative site. The mask may be objectionable to the patient and can interfere with treatment in the anterior maxilla. The level of sedation relies heavily on psychological reassurance and the ability of the dental surgeon to induce a semi-hypnotic state. The technique requires of the patient a certain level of understanding and compliance in terms of breathing through the nose, for this reason it is not suitable for very young children and some handicapped patients.

Safety and complications of relative analgesia

Relative analgesia sedation has an excellent safety record. To date there have been no recorded cases of significant morbidity or mortality occurring from relative analgesia in the United Kingdom. Provided that the dental surgeon is adequately trained, patients are carefully selected and the correct equipment with specific safety features is used, then relative analgesia is a very safe and effective technique for providing sedation, especially in children.

The principal complications associated with relative analgesia stem largely from the effects of over-sedation. A patient who is appropriately sedated should be able to readily maintain verbal contact, maintain a patent airway, swallow and keep his/her mouth and eyes open. An individual who is becoming over-sedated will have a glazed appearance, will persistently close his/her mouth and may complain of nausea and dizziness. If over-sedation is allowed to progress the patient will ultimately become unresponsive and may lose consciousness. The status of the patient must be closely monitored by the dental surgeon and dental nurse so that signs of over-sedation can be recognized as early as possible. If the patient starts to become over-sedated the nitrous oxide concentration should immediately be reduced by 10–20%, whereupon the patient should quickly become more alert.

Sometimes vomiting occurs during sedation with nitrous oxide. The incidence can be minimized first, by only sedating starved patients (> 2 hours), and second, by not over-sedating the patient. If a patient actually becomes unconscious (which should never happen), dental treatment should be immediately abandoned, the nitrous oxide should be switched off and 100% oxygen administered. The patient's airway must be maintained and, if necessary, ventilation should be supplemented, until consciousness is regained. Such occurrences are, fortunately, rare and are usually the result of undue hypersensitivity to nitrous oxide. It is salutary to remember that individual response to nitrous oxide, as to any drug, is subject to considerable variation.

Medical emergencies can arise during sedation or at any other time and are described fully in Chapter 8. Suffice it to say that the management of emergencies in children is a specialized field. In an emergency the clinical condition of a child can deteriorate very rapidly. It is essential that all dental surgeons providing relative analgesia for children should be trained in paediatric basic life support.

The remaining complications which can affect patients following relative analgesia are relatively minor. From a pharmacological point of view nitrous oxide should be completely eliminated from the body within minutes of the termination of sedation. However, some patients experience tiredness, amnesia and nausea in the hours following nitrous oxide administration presumably due to the general disturbance of their metabolism. The management of these sequelae is simply for the patient to rest quietly at home until the effect has completely resolved.

Finally, under the heading of complications, it is important to highlight the problem of chronic exposure of dental personnel to nitrous oxide. Studies have shown that long-term exposure to nitrous oxide may result in an increased incidence of liver, renal and neurological disease. There is evidence of bone marrow toxicity and interference with vitamin B_{12} synthesis which can lead to signs and symptoms similar to those of pernicious anaemia (see Chapter 4). There is a proven inhibitory effect of nitrous oxide on the reproductive system and an increased incidence of spontaneous abortion in women who have been chronically exposed to nitrous oxide.

The Health and Safety Commission in the United Kingdom have specified that dental staff should not be exposed to more than an average of 100 p.p.m. nitrous oxide over any 8-hour period. In order to achieve this level and keep nitrous oxide pollution to a minimum in the dental surgery there are a number of recommendations to be followed. First, scavenging equipment must be used. Active scavenging involves the removal of waste gases by the application of low power suction to the expiratory limb of the breathing circuit (Figure 5.11). Passive scavenging includes measures such as opening a window or door, using a fan to improve surgery ventilation, and extending the expiratory limb so that

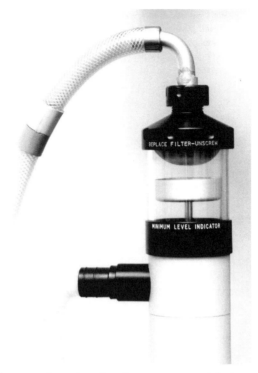

Figure 5.11 An active scavenging system where the gases are evacuated using suction.

exhaled gas is voided outside the building or surgery area. The main cause of pollution from relative analgesia is leakage of gas from around the nose mask and mouth breathing. There is a legal requirement for dental surgeons to comply with health and safety regulations. All steps should be taken to minimize unnecessary staff exposure to nitrous oxide. Pregnant women and those trying to conceive should not be allowed to work in a surgery where nitrous oxide is being used.

Despite all the precautions required and the skill needed in using relative analgesia, it is a technique which is tried and tested and one which most patients find helpful in managing mild anxiety. Its use is likely to remain more popular in children since, as with oral sedatives, relative analgesia offers most patients a non-threatening approach to sedation.

References and further reading

Crawford, A.N. (1990). The use of nitrous oxide-oxygen inhalational sedation with local analgesia as an alternative to general anaesthesia for dental extractions in children. *British Dental Journal*, **168**, 395–398.

Donaldson, D. and Meechan, J.G. (1995). The hazards of chronic exposure to nitrous oxide: an update. *British Dental Journal*, **178**, 95–100.

Health and Safety Commission (1995). *Anaesthetic Agents: Controlling Exposure under COSHH*. London: HMSO.

Roberts, G.J. (1990). Inhalational sedation (relative analgesia) with oxygen/nitrous oxide gas mixtures. 1. Principles. *Dental Update*, **17**, 139–146.

Roberts, G.J. (1990). Inhalational sedation (relative analgesia) with oxygen/nitrous oxide gas mixtures. 2. Practical techniques. *Dental Update*, **17**, 190–196.

6

Intravenous sedation: principles and practice

Introduction

Intravenous sedation is the technique of choice for most adult dental patients undergoing conscious sedation. The administration of sedation agents via the intravenous route normally produces a predictable and reliable pharmacological effect. Intravenous sedation is more potent and quicker acting than inhalational or oral sedation and is particularly effective for very anxious or phobic dental patients and for difficult surgical procedures. It produces true pharmacological sedation rather than psychopharmacological sedation that is achieved with inhalational techniques.

The practice of intravenous sedation is technique sensitive, especially in comparison with inhalational and oral sedation. It requires the ability to perform intravenous cannulation which, even for the experienced dentist, can be a difficult technique to master. The dental surgeon also has to be able to determine an appropriate end-point for sedation and drug administration. The level of sedation needs to be sufficient to enable the patient to accept operative dentistry but not so great as to present the risk of over-sedation.

The aim of this chapter is to provide the theoretical basis from which sound clinical principles and skilled practical techniques can be developed to ensure the safe practice of intravenous sedation. The material can only provide a didactic background to good practice. It is essential that supervised hands-on training and competency is achieved before applying these clinical techniques to patients.

Indications and contra-indications for intravenous sedation

Intravenous sedation is almost exclusively used for adult dental patients. It is particularly indicated for moderately to severely anxious or phobic dental patients. These individuals require powerful pharmacological sedation to overcome their fears and may even need some form of oral premedication prior to receiving intravenous sedation. Similarly, patients undergoing traumatic surgical procedures, such as third molar surgery or apicectomy, require a potent sedation technique which can normally only be achieved by intravenous agents. The amnesic effect of the intravenous benzodiazepines may be useful in negating the memory of traumatic dental procedures. The ability of intravenous benzodiaze-pines to inhibit the pharyngeal gag reflex means that intravenous sedation is particularly useful for patients who are unable to tolerate oral instrumentation.

Intravenous sedation is also indicated in patients who have mild medical conditions which may be aggravated by the stress of dental treatment. These include, for example, patients with mild hypertension or asthma. Careful assess-ment of these patients is required in order to establish the potential risk of sedation in relation to the medical condition and potential interactions with drug therapy. Intravenous sedation also has an important role in patients who are unable to co-operate fully. Such individuals often wish to receive dental care but because of their limited understanding or inability to keep still are unable to receive routine dentistry. Mild mental or physical handicap and cerebral dis-orders are the commonest conditions where intravenous sedation can be helpful.

Intravenous sedation has an important role in the management of patients with severe systemic disease or moderate to severe handicap, especially if it avoids the need for general anaesthesia. However, these patients do present a significant risk and intravenous sedation should only be undertaken in a specialist hospital environment. Intravenous sedation is contra-indicated where there is a history of allergy to benzodiazepines or if there has been a history of undue sensitivity to anaesthetic agents. This may be particularly relevant when there may be a family history of malignant hyperthermia (hyperpyrexia). Impaired renal or hepatic function interferes with the metabolism and excretion of virtually all drugs and, therefore, presents another contra-indication. It is also not advisable to use intravenous sedation during pregnancy and breast feeding and for patients with severe psychiatric disease or drug dependency.

Intravenous sedation is contra-indicated in severe needle phobics who are unable to accept any type of injection. Inhalational or oral sedation may be an acceptable alternative for these patients but sometimes it is necessary to com-bine two techniques. Inhalational sedation (or even hypnosis) may be employed initially to relax the patient enough to allow venous cannulation; once the cannula has been inserted the intravenous sedative can be administered and the inhalational element of the sedation switched off. Intravenous techniques are also, to some extent, contra-indicated in patients with poor veins. This includes patients with excessive subcutaneous fat whose veins are not visible and the elderly who frequently have friable veins which are prone to damage during cannulation.

The use of intravenous sedation in children should be approached with caution. Not only do children dislike needles but intravenous sedation agents can have an unpredictable effect. Children can lose their controlling inhibitions and become uncooperative. In the event of a complication, their condition can deteriorate very rapidly. Even slight over-sedation can result in significant respiratory depression and airway obstruction. Intravenous sedation in children should be undertaken only in very special circumstances and only by a specialist in sedation.

Drug choice for intravenous sedation

Intravenous sedation agents should not only have the ability to depress the central nervous system in order to produce a state of conscious sedation but they should also have a margin of safety wide enough to render the unintended loss of consciousness unlikely.

Modern intravenous sedation techniques depend almost exclusively on the benzodiazepines. Both midazolam and diazepam are suitable intravenous sedatives, although the pharmacokinetics of midazolam make this the preferred choice for dental sedation. Midazolam (trade name Hypnovel®) is presented in two concentrations: 2 mg/ml in a 5-ml ampoule and 5 mg/ml in a 2-ml ampoule. Although both presentations contain the same amount of midazolam, the 2 mg/ml (5-ml vial) formulation is less concentrated and easier to titrate because of the smaller volume required for the equivalent dose. Diazepam can be used to produce conscious sedation but its prolonged elimination and recovery time means that it is not ideal for short dental procedures.

Both midazolam and diazepam have the advantage of being reversible with flumazenil (Figure 6.1). In the past, other drugs have been used for intravenous sedation but whilst some have been termed sedative, most are really general anaesthetic agents used in smaller than usual doses, with a very fine margin of safety. These drugs have included agents such as pentobarbitone, pethidine and scopolamine (the Jorgensen technique), thiopentone and methohexitone. The use of these agents for intravenous sedation by dental surgeons is no longer a safe or acceptable practice and they should only be used by trained anaesthetists with access to specialist facilities.

New intravenous agents are currently undergoing clinical trials to evaluate their application to dental sedation. The most promising new agent is propofol, a short-acting anaesthetic drug administered via a continuous infusion. It has an extremely rapid recovery period which is very advantageous for ambulatory patients. It has been the subject of some quite extensive trials and its properties do offer several potential benefits particularly with reference to patient-controlled sedation (PCS, see p. 93).

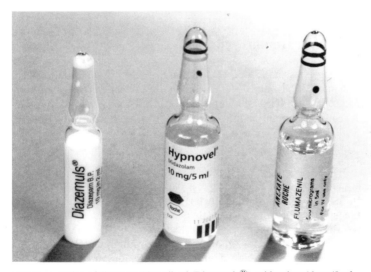

Figure 6.1 Presentation of diazepam 10 mg/2 ml (Diazemuls®), midazolam 10 mg/5 ml (Hypnovel®) and flumazenil 500 μg/5 ml (Anexate®).

Clinical effects of sedation with intravenous midazolam

Midazolam provides conscious sedation with acute detachment (lack of awareness of one's surroundings) for a period of 20–30 minutes after administration, followed by a period of relaxation which may last for a further hour or more. It produces some anterograde amnesia, that is loss of memory following administration of the drug. It also causes muscle relaxation and has an anticonvulsant action, so it is useful for sedating patients with cerebral disorders or epilepsy respectively. It only produces slight cardiovascular and respiratory depression when it is administered by a technique of slow, incremental intravenous injection. Midazolam has a reasonably wide margin of safety between the end point of sedation and loss of consciousness or anaesthesia although it is easy to induce sleep with moderate over-dosage. A satisfactory level of sedation is attained pharmacologically rather than psychologically. Recovery occurs within a reasonable period and the patient can usually be discharged home less than two hours following completion of treatment.

Although midazolam is the best agent currently available for intravenous sedation for dental procedures, it does have a number of disadvantages. It may alter a patient's perception and response to pain but it does not produce any clinically useful analgesia. For a short period after injection the laryngeal reflexes may be obtunded and overdosage may result in profound respiratory depression, particularly in patients with impaired respiratory function or in those who have taken other depressants, such as alcohol. Excessively rapid intravenous injection can also cause significant respiratory depression and even apnoea. Because of this risk, some authorities have suggested that supplemental oxygen should always be administered although this has yet to gain wide acceptance. Finally, intravenous midazolam may occasionally produce disinhibition, so instead of becoming more relaxed the patient becomes more anxious and difficult to manage.

Planning for intravenous sedation

Careful planning is essential before undertaking intravenous sedation in dental practice. Chapter 3 has already dealt with the selection and assessment of patients for sedation. The following sections will specify the personnel and equipment required to practice intravenous sedation both safely and effectively.

Personnel

Dental surgeons should not undertake sedation unless they have been appropriately trained. In the UK this means that dentists should have received relevant post-graduate training. This involves completing a recognized course which provides both didactic and clinical training in conscious sedation techniques. It is acceptable for an appropriately trained dental surgeon both to sedate the patient and to provide dental treatment simultaneously. However, as a minimum requirement the dental surgeon must be assisted by a dental nurse or other person who is appropriately trained and who is capable of monitoring the clinical condition of the patient. It is also essential that all staff are trained to assist in the event of an emergency. The dental nurse must be specifically trained in sedation and resuscitation techniques as this is not part of the core training for dental nurses.

Equipment

The suitability of the dental surgery where sedation is provided needs to be assessed. Easy access and space for patients, staff and for the management of emergencies is required. There should be the facility to store sedation agents and other drugs in a locked drugs cupboard. The dental chair must have a fast-recline mechanism so that in an emergency the patient can be quickly laid supine. There should be a high volume aspirator available (with emergency back-up) which can be used to clear the oropharynx.

The dental surgery must be prepared with equipment for monitoring the patient's clinical condition during sedation. A pulse oximeter is mandatory to measure continuously oxygen saturation and heart rate. A manual or automatic sphygmomanometer is required to monitor baseline blood pressure before sedation and, if required, during sedation. Emergency equipment and drugs, as detailed in Chapter 8, must also be available. It is particularly important to have the facility to provide supplemental oxygen via a nasal cannula or a face mask, and a device with which to give positive pressure ventilation. The emergency equipment required for sedation is identical to that which should be stocked in any dental practice; the only additional item required for undertaking benzodiazepine sedation is the reversal agent, flumazenil (trade name Anexate®). This is presented as a clear liquid in 500-μg ampoules.

Ideally there should be a separate recovery area where the patient can sit quietly and privately following sedation. Oxygen and a suction apparatus must be available in the recovery area. An alternative is to allow the patient to recover in the dental chair but this ties up the chair for several hours and may not be possible in a busy dental practice.

Specific items of sedation equipment are required to administer intravenous drugs (Figure 6.2). Disposable 5-ml graduated syringes and 21-gauge hypodermic needles are needed to draw up the intravenous drugs. A tourniquet, surgical wipes and adhesive tape (or proprietary dressings) are required for venepuncture. It is preferable to establish venous access using an indwelling Teflonated cannula rather than a butterfly needle. A Teflonated cannula provides more secure access and is less likely to become dislodged or blocked during limb movement. A 22-gauge cannula is the ideal size for administering intravenous sedation. It readily allows the administration of modest volumes of drugs but is small enough not to cause too much discomfort on insertion.

Technique of intravenous sedation

Pre-procedural checks

The patient scheduled for intravenous sedation should have undergone thorough pre-operative assessment as described in Chapter 3. The availability of appro-

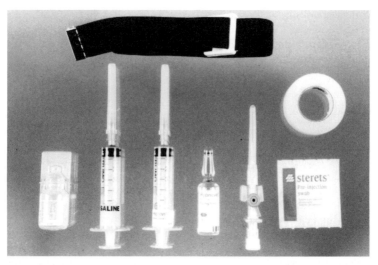

Figure 6.2 Equipment required for the administration of intravenous sedation agents: tourniquet, adhesive tape, surgical wipes, 22-gauge cannula, two 5-ml syringes and 21-gauge needles, ampoules of saline and sedation drug.

priate personnel and equipment should be checked before the start of each sedation session. It is helpful to use a pre-procedural checklist such as the one illustrated in Figure 6.3. This ensures that all the necessary criteria required to practise sedation safely are confirmed before the start of the session. Each item on the list should be checked and the appropriate box ticked. Equipment should not only be available but also in good working order. Gas cylinders and particularly oxygen supplies must be checked to ensure that they contain a sufficient volume of gas and are not empty. The expiry date on all drugs should be checked to ensure that they are still valid.

Before the patient arrives in the dental surgery all the equipment required for the session should be prepared and placed discretely out of the patient's line of vision. The patient is then brought into the surgery and seated in the dental chair. It is important to keep waiting time to a minimum, as delays only increase the fear of an already anxious patient. The procedure for sedation and the dental treatment to be performed on that visit should be briefly re-explained to the patient. The records should be consulted to ensure that written consent has been obtained. Medical and drug history should be re-confirmed, in particular asking about any changes since the assessment appointment. The time of the last meal and drink should be sought; a minimum of two hours starvation is required. Finally, the dental surgeon should be sure that the patient has a suitable escort to care for them after the treatment appointment and confirm that appropriate transport is available. The patient history forms part of the pre-procedural checklist shown in Figure 6.3. Before any sedation procedure is commenced the blood pressure should be taken and a pulse oximeter probe attached to the patient's finger or ear lobe. Once they are seated comfortably the chair can be reclined in preparation for venepuncture.

PRE-SEDATION CHECKLIST

Patient's Name	Date of Birth	Record Number

Date	
Dental surgeon	
1st Dental nurse	
2nd Dental nurse	

1. Staff Check:	
Experienced qualified dental nurse present?	
Another dental surgeon or nurse within easy call?	
Dental surgeon & nurse know emergency procedure?	
2. Emergency & Monitoring Equipment Check:	
Site of emergency equipment known	
Oxygen - emergency/routine	
Suction - mobile-back up/dental unit	
Positive pressure ventilating bag	
Sphygmomanometer - manual/automatic	
Pulse oximeter	
Emergency drugs available and in date	
Flumazenil	
3. Sedation Equipment Check:	
Midazolam, sodium chloride (drug, conc^n, exp date)	
22g cannulae, 5ml syringes, green needles, drug labels (x2)	
Tourniquet, alcohol wipe, micropore tape, watch with second hand	
4. Patient Check:	
Patient/parent understands what is planned	
Written consent obtained	
Medical history checked	
Normal medication taken	
Last meal/drink (Fasting-give glucose) (Alcohol-postpone)	
Escort & transport	

Figure 6.3 Pre-sedation checklist.

Venepuncture and intravenous cannulation

Establishing intravenous access is essential to the success of intravenous sedation. An indwelling cannula, which is present throughout the period of sedation and recovery, is mandatory to safe sedation practice. It is not acceptable simply to inject an intravenous sedation agent using a syringe and needle, which is then removed once the drug has been administered. Venous access is required not only for the administration of the sedation agent but also, in the event of an emergency, for the administration of a reversal agent or other emergency drug. Untoward occurrences can occur at any time during the treatment appointment so it is essential that once venous access has been established the cannula should remain in situ until the patient is finally discharged home.

Venous access has traditionally been achieved using a butterfly needle, which is relatively easy to insert. This technique has a number of disadvantages which include irritation of the vein wall by the metallic needle, clotting and obstruction of the lumen of the needle, dislodgement of the needle and tissuing caused by limb movement. More recently the teflonated cannula has superseded the use of the butterfly needle. Insertion of cannulae is more technique-sensitive but the venous access obtained is far more secure. Teflon® is non-irritant to veins and, due to its low adhesive surface, the cannula rarely blocks during short procedures. In addition it can bend during limb movement and once in place it will rarely become dislodged.

There are two main sites of venous access for the purposes of dental sedation; the dorsum of the hand and the antecubital fossa. The dorsum of the hand has a variable network of veins (Figure 6.4) which drain into the cephalic and basilic veins of the forearm (Figure 6.5). These veins provide the first choice for establishing venous access. They are accessible, superficial, readily visible, stabilized by the underlying bones of the hand and are distant from vital structures. The disadvantage of the dorsal veins of the hand is that they are poorly tethered and tend to move during the insertion of a cannula. Movement can be minimized by stretching the skin and inserting the cannula into a

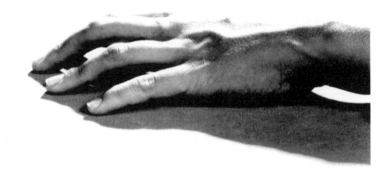

Figure 6.4 Venous network of the dorsum of the hand.

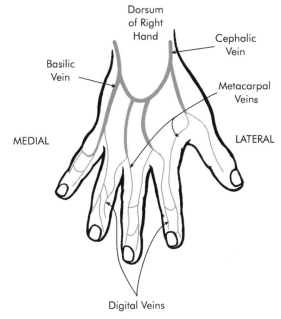

Figure 6.5 Superficial venous anatomy of the dorsum of the hand.

bifurcation where two veins join together. The dorsal veins of the hand are also subject to peripheral vasoconstriction in cold weather and in patients who are very anxious. Vasoconstriction can usually be reversed by warming the hand in a bowl of warm water prior to venepuncture. In addition the back of the hand is somewhat painful to puncture and consideration should be given to using a topical application of local anaesthetic such as Ametop® or EMLA®. Topical sprays of ethyl chloride or other highly volatile substances should be avoided as they cause vasoconstriction and have the potential to cause skin necrosis due to the effect of frostbite.

The second choice for venous access is in the larger veins of the antecubital fossa (Figure 6.6). Here the two main veins of the forearm, the cephalic and basilic veins, pass the lateral and medial aspects of the antecubital fossa respectively. A further vein (the median vein) originates in the deep tissue of the forearm and divides to join the cephalic and basilic veins at the antecubital fossa. Any of these veins can be used for establishing venous access.

However, it is important to note that the brachial artery and the median nerve also pass through the antecubital fossa on its inner aspect, medial to the biceps tendon. Venepuncture and cannulation should ideally be restricted to the lateral aspect of the antecubital fossa, using the cephalic or median cephalic veins, in order to avoid accidental damage to vital structures. The antecubital fossa has the advantage of having veins which are usually large and well tethered. If not readily visible they can usually be palpated. Veins which are readily palpable but not particularly visible may be easier to cannulate than highly visual superficial veins. If necessary a line can be drawn on the skin surface lateral to the vein to identify its direction and thereby aid venepuncture.

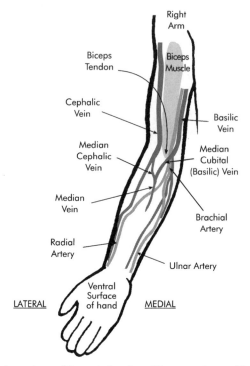

Figure 6.6 Vascular anatomy of the ventral surface of the arm and antecubital fossa.

The main disadvantage of the antecubital fossa is the proximity of important structures and the movement that occurs at the elbow joint. The use of an arm board to maintain an extended arm is sometimes necessary if the patient is unable to keep it straight themselves.

If veins are not suitable on either the dorsum of the hand or the antecubital fossa then the patient should be referred to a specialist. It is possible to utilize the large cephalic vein lateral to the radial artery as it runs from the wrist over the radius or the great saphenous vein of the foot as it passes over the medial malleolus. However, these veins are not really suitable for the inexperienced practitioner.

The key to successful venepuncture and cannulation is careful preparation of the site and a well-practised technique. Many dental surgeons see venepuncture as the most difficult part of the sedation technique to master. It is recommended that practitioners gain practical experience on mannequin arms or on willing colleagues before attempting to cannulate anxious patients who are unlikely to tolerate multiple unsuccessful attempts at venepuncture.

The patient should always be laid supine to minimize the chance of a vasovagal attack during venepuncture and to maximize the venous return from the extremities. A suitable vein should be selected and a tourniquet is placed about 10 cm above that site. The dental surgeon should then wait until the vein starts to become tense and filled with blood, which may take one or two minutes. The process can be accelerated by repeated clenching of the fist, thereby pumping blood into the obtunded vein. Gentle tapping of the skin over the vein often helps to make it more prominent, a process sometimes referred to as superficialization. Lowering the limb below the level of the heart will also increase venous filling.

With difficult veins, it may be possible to get better filling by using a sphygmomanometer cuff inflated to midway between diastolic and systolic pressure. Hot towels can also be applied to the skin to encourage vasodilatation. Adequate preparation of the vein is the key to successful venepuncture and only when the vein is sufficiently full should venepuncture be attempted.

The skin should be cleaned with water or a suitable antiseptic such as isopropyl alcohol. The latter tends to cause pain on injection unless it has completely evaporated and there is no scientific evidence that the use of alcohol is of any real benefit. The skin is then tensed and the cannula inserted at an angle of around 10–15° (Figure 6.7). It is passed through the skin and into the underlying vein for a distance of around 1 cm. Skilful phlebotomists view venepuncture as a two-stage process initially penetrating the skin and subsequently the vein. A small flashback of blood indicates correct localization of the cannula in the lumen of the vein. If no flashback is seen then the cannula is still in the subcutaneous tissues and needs to be carefully advanced forward or laterally through the vein wall. Once a flashback of blood is visible the Teflon part of the cannula is advanced up to its hub, leaving the insertion needle static (Figure 6.8). It is better to move the Teflonated section forward rather than the needle backwards as this runs a greater risk of the cannula becoming extravenous. Finally, the needle is removed completely and a cap is removed from it so that it can be placed on the aperture of the cannula (Figure 6.9). To avoid blood spilling onto the patient pressure should be applied just proximal to the vein where the cannula is situated. Finally, the extravenous section of the cannula is fixed securely in place using non-allergenic surgical tape or proprietary dressing.

The correct positioning and patency of the cannula may be tested by

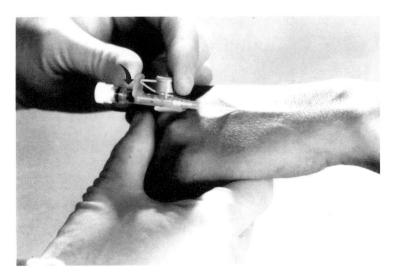

Figure 6.7 Technique of intravenous cannulation. The cannula is inserted through the skin at an angle of 10–15° and advanced into the underlying vein. A small flashback of blood (marked with arrow) confirms that the cannula is in the lumen of the vein.

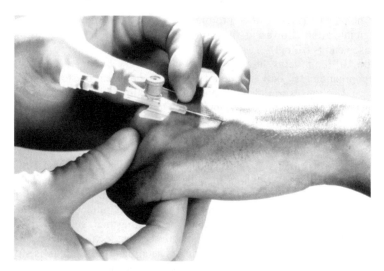

Figure 6.8 The Teflon cannula is advanced over the metal insertion needle into the vein. The metal needle should remain static as the cannula is advanced forward.

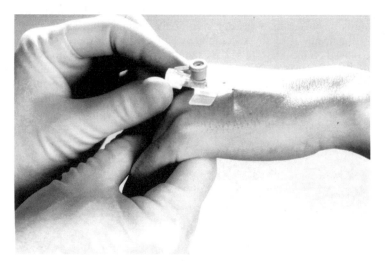

Figure 6.9 Once the cannula is fully inserted the metal needle is removed and a cap is placed on the distal aperture of the cannula.

administering 2–3 ml of 0.9% saline intravenously (Figure 6.10). If the cannula is sited in the lumen of the vein the saline will pass easily into the general circulation. In contrast, if the cannula has come out of the vein and is in the subcutaneous tissues, the saline will pool and a small lump will appear under the skin. If this happens the cannula should be removed and reinserted at another site. The patient may feel a cold sensation moving up the arm when saline is administered into a correctly positioned cannula. If, however, there is a complaint of pain radiating down the arm, the injection must be stopped as this indicates accidental arterial cannulation.

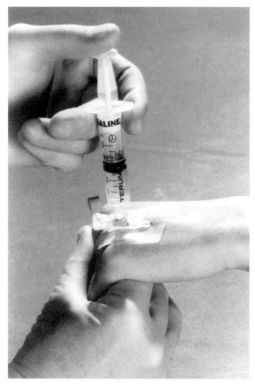

Figure 6.10 A test dose of 0.9% saline is administered to confirm the position and patency of the cannula.

Titration of sedation agent

The syringe containing the prepared drug (usually midazolam 10 mg in 5 ml) is attached to the delivery port of the cannula (Figure 6.11). The patient is warned that he/she will begin to feel relaxed and sleepy over the next 10 minutes. The first increment of 1 mg (0.5 ml) midazolam is injected slowly over 15 seconds, followed by a pause for 1 minute. Further doses of 1 mg are delivered, with an interval of 1 minute between increments, until the level of sedation is judged to be adequate. The aim of intravenous sedation is to titrate incremental doses of drug according to the patient's response (Figure 6.12). The dental surgeon should keep talking to the patient whilst carefully watching for the effects of sedation as well as any adverse reactions, especially respiratory depression. The sedation end-point is reached when several specific signs of sedation are apparent. These signs include:

1. slurring and slowing of speech;
2. relaxed demeanour;
3. delayed response to commands;
4. willingness to undergo treatment;
5. positive EVE's sign (see below);
6. Verrill's sign (see below).

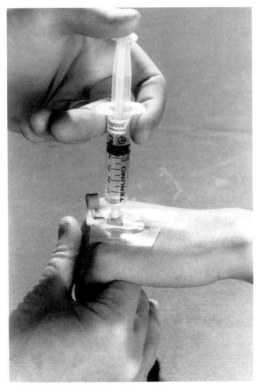

Figure 6.11 Administration of sedation agent—midazolam.

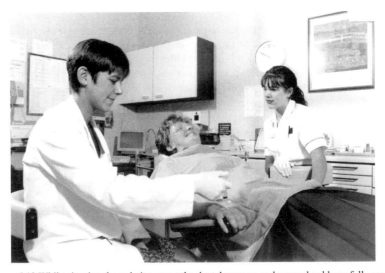

Figure 6.12 Whilst titrating the sedation agent the dental surgeon and nurse should carefully monitor the patient.

The EVE sign is a test of motor co-ordination. Patients are requested to touch the tip of their nose with a finger. A sedated patient will be unable to perform this simple task accurately and usually touches the top lip (Figure 6.13).

Verrill's sign occurs when there is ptosis or drooping of the upper eyelid, to an extent that it lies approximately half way across the pupil (Figure 6.14). This is a variable sign which is more common with intravenous diazepam than with midazolam and may represent an early sign of over-sedation with midazolam. However, the signs of sedation are not exclusive and often only two or three are present to different degrees in any one indi- vidual. They do, however, give some objective indication of an adequate level of sedation.

The essential criterion for conscious sedation is that communication is maintained with the patient and that they will respond to the clinician's instructions. Determining an appropriate end-point for sedation is often difficult but depends on the ability of the dental surgeon to recognize specific signs and to maintain rapport with the patient. There is considerable variation in the dose required to produce adequate sedation between individual patients, and even between different sessions for the same patient. Factors such as the extent of dental fear, concurrent drug therapy, the amount of sleep the previous night and the level of stress at home are so variable that it is impossible to predict how much drug will be required for a specific patient on a certain day. This is why careful titration of the dose of sedation agent, in response to specific signs, is so important for the practice of safe sedation. If drug dose was to be based on weight only then numerous patients would become either over- or under- sedated. When the patient is judged to be appropriately sedated the syringe containing the sedation drug is removed. No further increments of drug are given when a standardized technique is adopted.

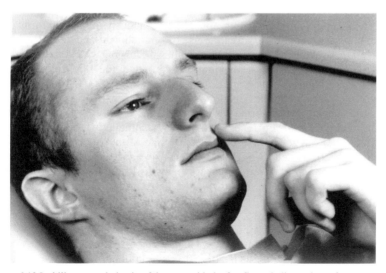

Figure 6.13 Inability to touch the tip of the nose with the forefinger indicates loss of motor co-ordination and is known as EVE's sign.

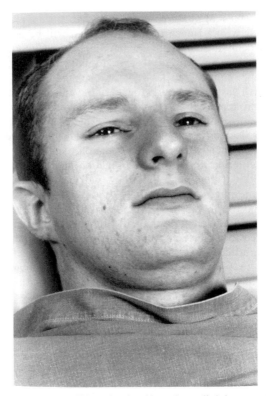

Figure 6.14 Ptosis of the upper eyelids so that they bisect the pupils is known as Verrill's sign.

Clinical and electromechanical monitoring

The clinical condition of the patient must be continuously monitored throughout the sedation session. This involves the use of both clinical and electromechanical techniques. Clinical monitoring includes reviewing the patency of the patient's airway, the pattern of respiration, the pulse, the skin colour and the patient's responsiveness. These signs must be observed on a continuous basis by the dental surgeon and by the dental nurse.

Electromechanical monitoring should include both pulse oximetry and blood pressure measurement. Pulse oximetry is a technique which measures the patient's arterial oxygen saturation and pulse rate from a probe attached to the finger or ear lobe (Figure 6.15). The oximeter works by measuring and comparing the absorption of two different wavelengths of red and infra-red light by the blood. The colour of the blood changes according to the degree of oxygen saturation and this in turn affects the absorption spectrum. By calculating the relative absorption of the two wavelengths the oximeter can calculate oxygen saturation very precisely. The pulse oximeter is accurate to approximately 1%, a vast improvement on the human eye which cannot detect skin colour change until the oxygen saturation falls by 10–20%. In addition the pulse oximeter will be accurate in patients who are anaemic when the clinical signs of cyanosis are even more difficult to detect.

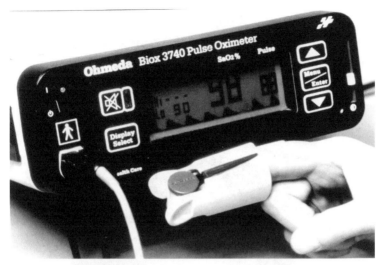

Figure 6.15 The pulse oximeter measures the patient's arterial oxygen saturation and heart rate from a probe attached to the finger or ear lobe.

Oxygen saturation is an excellent monitor of both respiratory and cardio-vascular function. Patients undergoing sedation should always have an oxygen saturation well above 90%. If the saturation drops below this level it is an indication of inhibited respiratory or cardiovascular activity. The cause should be promptly investigated and corrected. The most common causes of oxygen desaturation during sedation are slight respiratory depression, breath holding or over-sedation. The problem is usually rectified by asking the patient to take a few deep breaths. If the saturation remains below 90%, oxygen should be administered via a nasal cannula at a rate of 2–4 litres/min (Figure 6.16). If the patient's saturation still does not rise then the most likely cause is over-sedation. In such cases the sedation should be reversed with flumazenil.

The pulse oximeter is essentially an early warning device. It will indicate an initial problem which, with swift intervention, can be corrected before the situation becomes more serious. However, it should be remembered that the pulse oximeter is not infallible. Correct functioning of the equipment can be affected by excessive movement, pigmented skin, nail varnish and fluorescent or bright lights. Aberrant values should always be confirmed by clinical observation of the patient. Pulse oximeters have an audible alarm which is activated when the saturation or pulse rate drops below a specific threshold. For routine intravenous sedation the alarm should be set to sound if the saturation drops below 90% or the pulse goes below 50 or above 120. Bradycardia may indicate a vasovagal attack, vagal stimulation or hypoxia. Tachycardia usually results from inadequate analgesia and pain control. Any values outside the accepted range should result in immediate cessation of dental treatment followed by investigation and prompt rectification of the cause.

Continuous monitoring of blood pressure throughout sedation is not necessary. The blood pressure should be taken immediately before intravenous sedation is administered, to provide a baseline value. Most hypertensive patients will have been identified at the assessment appointment and referred for medical

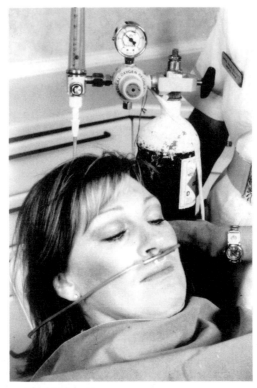

Figure 6.16 Supplemental oxygen can be conveniently administered via a nasal cannula. The nasal cannula can also be used with nitrous oxide sedation when it allows better access to the mouth, especially in the upper incisor region.

opinion. Some elevation of blood pressure is to be expected in anxious dental patients but if values are excessive (more than 160/95) then sedation should be postponed until a later date. The blood pressure needs only to be repeated during treatment if there is a concern over the clinical condition of the patient or in the event of an emergency. Blood pressure can be taken by using either a manual sphygmomanometer or by an automatic blood pressure machine.

It should be remembered that simple observation of the patient's clinical status is the most important type of monitoring. Although pulse oximetry is mandatory it should not detract the dental surgeon and the dental nurse from continuously assessing the patient's clinical condition.

Dental treatment

The administration of local analgesia and start of operative dentistry can begin as soon as the patient has reached the appropriate level of sedation. Approximately 30–40 minutes of operating time is usually available and treatment should be planned so that it can be readily completed in this time. It is good practice to undertake traumatic procedures, such as bone removal and cavity preparation, at the beginning of the session while the patient is in a state of acute detachment. After 30–40 minutes the effect of sedation starts to wear off and co-operation may be reduced. This is the time to concentrate on simple procedures such as suturing or carving restorations.

Intravenous sedation using a single benzodiazepine produces no analgesia, so it is essential to provide effective pain control during dental procedures. This should include the use of both topical analgesia and sufficient quantities of local anaesthetic. Sedated patients will still respond to pain, although their response will be reduced. The muscle relaxant effect of sedation makes it difficult for patients to keep their mouths open during treatment. A mouth prop can improve access for the dental surgeon and make treatment more comfortable for the patient. It must never be an excuse, however, for failing to maintain conversation with patients and checking that their responses to instructions remain intact.

During sedation the gag reflex is significantly diminished and immediately following drug administration the laryngeal reflexes may also be reduced. The airway must be protected from any obstruction and this is best achieved by high volume aspiration. When small instruments are used, butterfly sponge or a rubber dam must be inserted to protect against foreign bodies accidentally falling back into the airway. Great care should be exercised when extracting teeth in the sedated patient. Use of a tongue retractor and good suction will help to prevent segments of crowns, roots or amalgam entering the pharynx.

Recovery

At the end of the dental procedure the patient is slowly returned to the upright position over a period of several minutes. They are then transferred to the recovery area and seated in a comfortable chair. Patients should not be moved from the dental chair until they can walk with minimal assistance. Whilst in the recovery area patients should be under the direct supervision of the dental team or their escorts.

At least one hour should have elapsed since the last increment of drug was administered before patients can be discharged. They must not be discharged until sufficiently recovered so as to be able to stand and walk without assistance. When the dental surgeon determines that patients are ready to leave they should be discharged into the care of their escort who must be given full verbal and written instructions about their postoperative care (Figure 6.17). The patient should rest quietly at home for the rest of the day and refrain from driving, drinking alcohol and operating machinery or domestic appliances for 24 hours.

The venous cannula should remain *in situ* until just before the patient is discharged. It should be taken out by carefully removing the surgical tape or dressing and withdrawing the cannula (Figure 6.18). Firm pressure is then maintained with a cotton wool roll on the venepuncture site for several minutes to prevent haematoma formation. If significant bleeding occurs when the cannula is removed it can also be helpful to elevate the arm for a period of two to three minutes.

Patient-controlled sedation

The technique of patient-controlled sedation (PCS) was adapted from that of patient-controlled analgesia (PCA) which has become widely accepted as a

AFTER YOUR SEDATION

- You should go home with your escort and rest quietly for the remainder of the day.

- You must not drink any alcoholic drinks for the next 24 hours.

- You must not operate any machinery, attempt to drive or sign anything important for the next 24 hours.

- Please take any medicines you have been prescribed. (*always read the label!*).

- Don't worry if you have difficulty remembering what has happened today. This is called 'amnesia' and is very common.

- Please telephone us if you have any problems or queries at all.

Your next appointment will be on ....

at.................. to see.............................

Figure 6.17 An example of written instructions regarding postoperative care following sedation. The instructions should be reinforced verbally to patients and their escort.

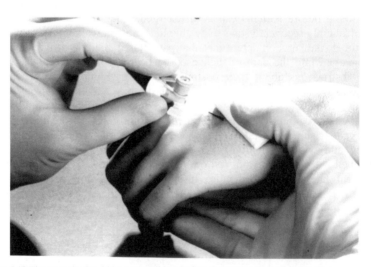

Figure 6.18 The cannula should be removed just before the patient is discharged. Firm pressure should be applied with a cotton wool roll after the cannula is removed to prevent the formation of a haematoma. If any bleeding occurs, the arm should be elevated to minimize the risk of bruising.

means of very satisfactorily controlling postoperative pain. PCS is an entirely logical step since operator determined levels of sedation may easily differ from the perceived need of the patient. As with the relief of pain, the patient is uniquely positioned to make the judgement as to the level of sedation required. It also helps to obviate the need to assess the depth of a patient's sedation from signs which are not always easy to determine. PCS has other advantages too: it will allow an incremental technique with little risk of overdosage and it can be less demanding on recovery time since it can be shown that patients will frequently administer themselves lower doses than clinicians would.

In order to understand why PCS is effective it is necessary to reiterate some of the pharmacological principles referred to earlier. The single injection (bolus injection) undergoes rapid dilution within seconds of administration and, coupled with variable circulation times, the delay before it has any effect on the central nervous system varies from 1 to 4 minutes. If small multiple doses are given, the result is a slightly slower build up of the plasma concentration but not as much as would be anticipated since a steady state is reached. After this has been achieved only small supplemental doses are required to maintain the level of sedation. Thus, for the technique to be effective, it is usually necessary to give a loading dose either by means of a single bolus or by more frequently repeated increments than are subsequently used.

The other factor that has made PCS a realistic prospect for future practice is the development of the microprocessor-controlled infusion pumps or syringes (Figure 6.19). These are both reliable and accurate and require the dentist to set only the required dose and the 'lock-out' period. The lock-out period (when the machine will not respond to the patient's prompts) also includes the infusion rate which can be altered from the standard measurements. This allows considerable variation in the ways in which drugs can be delivered, thereby adding further to the flexibility of the system. On the negative side, care must always be taken not to set the doses administered at a level which renders the unintended loss of

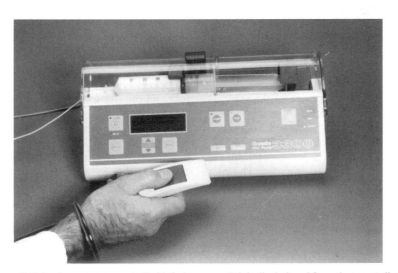

Figure 6.19 A microprocessor-controlled infusion pump. Originally designed for patient-controlled analgesia, these pumps can be adapted for use in patient-controlled sedation.

consciousness likely. However, providing the doses are set reasonably this should not pose too great a problem since the patient is unlikely to be able to press the control button if they are feeling too drowsy.

Current research using PCS techniques has been very promising. At the current time the syringe pumps are adapted from PCA systems and no specific PCS pump is available. All the published research to date has also been restricted to midazolam and propofol; other agents do not appear to have been tested. The great advantage of propofol, however, is its rapid metabolism which thus prevents the likelihood of accumulating high plasma concentrations of the drug with a consequently delayed recovery time.

Reversible sedation

Modern general anaesthesia relies heavily on using reversible techniques which provide excellent anaesthesia of variable duration followed by very rapid reversal at the end of the procedure. It seems entirely logical that sedation techniques should be based on a similar principle and yet the only drug, flumazenil, which would be suitable for this has not been accepted for such usage. This is partly due to the short half-life of the drug which renders a theoretical risk of re-sedation after reversal and partly due to the cost of the agent. In addition, the experience of sudden awakening after benzodiazepine sedation is also unpleasant. Even so, the prospect of developing reversible sedation is still realistic and it has been partly achieved with the use of PCS techniques like the one described above. A reliable reversal agent would represent a great step forwards but the costs of developing new drugs is prohibitively expensive and unlikely to occur unless there is a clear sustainable demand for new products.

Sedation records

Every sedation episode should be carefully documented in the patient notes. It can be helpful to use a printed sheet to record details of the sedation provided (Figure 6.20). The intravenous drug used, its expiry date and batch number should be noted, as well as the time of final increment and the total dose administered. The size of the venous cannula and the site where it was inserted should be recorded.

Although the patient is continuously monitored during sedation it is good practice to record the monitoring data at regular intervals. For the purposes of dental sedation the oxygen saturation, pulse and respiration rate should be recorded every 10 minutes. The more advanced pulse oximeters will do this automatically and provide a printout of the results. The dental treatment provided should also be documented in the normal way. At the end of the session a note should be made about the level of sedation and the operating conditions. This information will be useful when the patient re-attends for his/her next sedation appointment.

Finally, information about the recovery and discharge of the patient should be recorded. Assessment of the fitness of the patient for discharge, removal of the cannula, issue of postoperative instructions and discharge of the patient into the

SEDATION RECORD

Intravenous Drug	Expiry date	Batch Number	Time of Increments Initial Final	Total Dose Administered

Venous Access	Site	
	Cannula	

Monitoring Record

Time	Oxygen saturation	Pulse	Respiration rate	Blood pressure	Drugs/O_2, LA/ Oral procedure
Operative procedure undertaken					

Recovery and Discharge	
Recovery with escort/dental nurse	
Assessment of fitness for discharge	
Written post-sedation instructions to escort and patient	
Cannula removed	
Dental surgeon's approval to discharge	
Names of discharging - dental surgeon - dental nurse	
Time of discharge	

Signature of dental surgeon	

Figure 6.20 Sedation record sheet.

care of a responsible adult must all be documented. The record sheet should be attached to the patient notes along with the consent form so that there is a complete record of the treatment appointment.

Complications of intravenous sedation

The complications of sedation are discussed fully in Chapter 8 and are better avoided than confronted! Intravenous sedation is very safe provided that it is practised on carefully selected patients, in proper facilities, by appropriately-trained dental surgeons. The incidence of mortality associated with intravenous sedation in dentistry in the UK is extremely small. Potentially serious complications such as drug interactions, over-sedation, unconsciousness and respiratory depression are largely avoidable by careful patient selection and the use of a sound sedation technique.

Nevertheless, intravenous sedation does give rise to significant minor morbidity. Haematoma at the cannulation site, postoperative dizziness, nausea and headache are problems which affect a considerable number of patients. These relatively minor sequelae are difficult to avoid completely and are, for the most part, accepted side effects of either the sedation technique or the sedation agent. Patients should be warned of the possibility of such problems and dental surgeons should continually review their techniques to minimize the risk of any complication.

References and further reading

Dickenson, A.J. and Avery, B.S. (1995). A survey of in-dwelling intravenous cannula use in general dental practice. *British Dental Journal*, **179**, 89–92.

Oei-Lim, L.B., Vereulen-Cranch, D.M.E. and Bouvey-Berends, E.C.M. (1991). Conscious sedation with propofol in dentistry. *British Dental Journal*, **170**, 340–342.

Rosenbaum, N.R. and Hooper, P.A. (1988). The effects of flumazenil, a new benzodiazepine antagonist, on the reversal of midazolam sedation and amnesia in dental practice. *British Dental Journal*, **165**, 400–402.

Stephens, A.J. (1993). Intravenous sedation for handicapped dental patients: a clinical trial of midazolam and propofol. *British Dental Journal*, **179**, 89–92.

Ward, G.R. (1990). Intravenous sedation in general dental practice: why oximetry? *British Dental Journal*, **168**, 368–369.

7

Oral sedation and premedication

Introduction

Oral sedatives offer to most patients a non-threatening approach to sedation as they do not require injections and can be tried on a 'taste and see' basis. In addition to swallowing capsules or tablets, sedatives can also be given by rectal or nasal administration. Some of the latter methods are relatively new and in their early stages of development. They are mentioned here for the sake of completeness but it is too early to assess whether they will become commonly used although they are potentially useful in younger children.

The purpose of oral sedation and premedication is, to a large extent, the same but the use of premedication in an outpatient setting should be relatively rare. However, in both cases the principal purpose of the agent(s) is to alleviate fear and anxiety with a view to producing a relaxed, calm patient who can either tolerate further procedures or proceed to the induction of deeper sedation. In some circumstances the agents are used to diminish the response to pain rather than anxiety, either pre-operatively or postoperatively.

Oral sedation is a beneficial technique because it does not require any form of initial injection (which is obviously very useful for patients who are needle-phobic) and it is, without doubt, the simplest way of introducing the use of sedation into clinical practice. In many ways it can be considered more versatile than inhalational sedation since it does not require the same amount of patient co-operation in the initial stages. Most products are available in capsule, tablet or liquid formulations and can be dispensed as appropriate.

Requirements of oral sedatives

The ideal oral sedative would clearly fit the general criteria for sedation and would, therefore:

1. alleviate fear and anxiety;
2. not suppress protective reflexes;
3. be easy to administer;
4. be quickly effective;
5. be free of side effects;
6. be predictable in both duration and action;

7. be quickly metabolized and excreted;
8. not produce active metabolites;
9. have an active half-life of approximately 45–60 minutes.

It is clearly difficult to find any drug that fits all the above criteria and some of the features mentioned above are much easier to control in inhalational and intravenous sedation than they are with oral sedation. This is because of the variation in predictability that inevitably occurs in relation to:

1. an individual's degree of anxiety;
2. the pattern of absorption of the drug;
3. the rate of metabolism of the drug.

This leads to considerable individual variation in response which means that the outcome of many oral sedatives is less predictable than agents (even of the same chemical formulation) that are given parenterally. Despite this, oral sedatives have considerable advantages, the most obvious being that for most patients they are well tolerated and that they avoid the need for initial injections. In addition, their effect is usually longer lasting, although it may be less profound, than the same drug given intravenously.

There is a further advantage to oral premedication/sedation and that is that it can often be effective in overcoming the type of severe unreasoned behaviour (see Chapter 1) that may sometimes be encountered in the first 10–15 years of life. Such children rarely respond well to behavioural management techniques and no amount of explanation will produce co-operative behaviour in children exhibiting severe irrationality. However, even in such cases the purpose of sedation and premedication should be to introduce patients back to the practice of dentistry and to try and overcome their irrational behaviour over a period of time.

In adult patients, oral sedation is also helpful in overcoming fear and anxiety, whether rational or irrational. Geoffrey Foreman in 1974 stated that 'Since its origins, dentistry has, more than any other of the health sciences, been intimately associated with anxiety, fear and pain'. The principal function of the oral sedative is not actually to produce sedation; it is rather to provide anxiolysis. Similarly its main purpose is not to reduce pain, although if it does exhibit analgesic effects (as is the case with inhalational sedation) this could be regarded as beneficial. The fundamental objective when giving sedation should be a long-term aim of breaking the 'dentistry = pain' association described by Foreman, thereby allowing patients access to dental care which they would not otherwise tolerate.

It should be emphasized at this point that the purpose of sedation is **not** to produce a semi-comatose patient on whom large quantities of inadequate work can be quickly performed. It is regrettable that this may sometimes have occurred historically but with improved knowledge of the techniques of sedation, hopefully this will no longer remain the case.

A clearly-focused approach towards oral sedation should help the practitioner to use oral sedatives when they are appropriate. In adults this is usually best justified when sedation is being used to break down the barriers of fear and anxiety in order to reintroduce the patient to good dental care and to establish dental health of the highest standard. In such cases, sedation is most useful in the earlier appointments and with skilful management and general reduction of doses administered, its decreased use should ultimately result in sedation becoming unnecessary.

In the management of children, oral sedation can also be used to overcome behaviour resulting from previous bad experiences. These experiences can be either first or second-hand since they are extremely susceptible to parental expression. There is little doubt that the influence of parents on children's behaviour has a significant effect and that successful parenthood will commonly produce a confident self-assured child who can react favourably to new and even potentially threatening situations.

Parents who themselves appear anxious or disinterested (often seen as a result of family breakdown) frequently seem to instil a feeling of fear and mistrust in the child which is extremely difficult for a dentist to overcome. In such cases a long-term relationship is difficult to build up, particularly within the limitations of the health service.

From the dentist's point of view, management of a child's behaviour is best established with confident, self-assured and sympathetic handling since children instinctively perceive weakness in authority on the part of the dentist and behave accordingly (badly). The dentist must, therefore, assess the demands he can make on a child and if instructions are given they must be complied with so that confidence is built up in the relationship. In achieving this, it is important to be directive rather than authoritarian. Once the situation occurs that a child makes more and more demands on the dentist the relationship inevitably breaks down and treatment is rarely completed in such circumstances.

At that stage the decision has to be made as to whether sedation should be used or on rare occasions whether force should be used. In such cases, this must always be with the consent and agreement with the parents and the dentist must be absolutely certain in his own mind that he is acting in the best interests of the child and with the complete and stated agreement of the parents. Such a situation should be extremely rare and avoided wherever possible.

Children passing through their teenage years generally become more rational and, therefore, more open to reason. There are still many exceptions to this rule, however, since fear frequently persists as a result of previous bad experiences in the younger years or as a result of hearing of such experiences from friends and family. This fear can frequently be treated by the use of anxiolytic drugs, such as the benzodiazepines, although relatively higher doses may be required.

Finally, there are some children where behavioural problems are simply due to naughtiness although this can be extremely difficult to distinguish from genuine fear in some cases. Naughty behaviour, however, is much more common in front of parents or relatives and will frequently resolve if the parents can be persuaded to leave the child. This type of behaviour can usually be allayed by consistent discipline but in children where anxiety is the prime cause of naughtiness, sedation is another useful tool in alleviating bad behaviour.

Oral sedatives

Until the late 1960s the use of prescribed oral sedation for dental treatment was relatively rare, although quite a large number of patients would attempt their own sedation (usually with the self-administered assistance of alcohol!) when they were extremely anxious. Unfortunately this often interfered with their required treatment and did not always produce the desired effect. Even in the hospital situation, patients receiving premeditation for general anaesthesia would frequently be given intramuscular injections rather than oral sedatives and it is only in recent times that this practice has largely been discontinued in favour of the use of orally administered drugs.

Some of the oral sedatives in current use are listed below with their various properties. The list is not in any way exhaustive or exclusive but the different pharmacological groups commonly used have been included. It is interesting to note that where intravenous sedation techniques have advanced considerably in the past 10–15 years there has been relatively little change in the use of oral sedation and this remains an area where considerable research could provide beneficial results both for patients and dentists.

The benzodiazepines

Diazepam

Until recently, diazepam was the most commonly and widely used of all sedatives. It is a member of the benzodiazepine family, a large group of drugs with varying anxiolytic, sedative and hypnotic effects (see Chapter 4). It is available in tablets of 2 mg, 5 mg and 10 mg and is fairly reliably absorbed from the gut, its effect becoming apparent after about 30 minutes. The correct dosage for each individual is not easy to calculate since several factors influence its action. In particular, it does appear to bear a relationship to the age of a patient, much higher (relative) dosages being required in children and adolescents. As with intravenous administration, the converse is true in the elderly and infirm. As a rough guide a dose between 0.1 and 0.25 mg/kg of body weight will produce adequate sedation and should be given 1 hour before surgery and following a light snack. If there is any possibility that anaesthesia rather than sedation will be required, then no food or liquid should be taken pre-operatively although a small sip of water may be consumed for the purpose of swallowing the pills.

Administration of a single dose of oral diazepam does give the operator the opportunity to form a baseline assessment on which further action may be taken. Too high a dosage will cause sleep, whilst inadequate dosage will result in an alert and still anxious patient; this does allow the opportunity to add further oral doses if time permits or to proceed to intravenous sedation if necessary. Potential side effects include dizziness, increased pain awareness, ataxia (difficulty in maintaining posture) and occasional respiratory depression. Prolonged post-operative drowsiness has also been reported.

Caution is necessary in administering diazepam to patients with obvious psychoses, neuromuscular disorders, respiratory, liver or kidney disease. Alcohol intake must be prohibited for a period of 24 hours before and after administration. Patients should not drive or operate machinery for 24 hours post-medication. As with intravenous diazepam, there is also some risk of some re-sedation after 2–3 days due to the production of active metabolites.

Oral diazepam has been found particularly useful in the treatment of patients with cerebral palsy, coupling it with intravenous injection in severe cases (use of intravenous diazepam is considered in Chapter 6). A rectal preparation is also available and this may be of use on rare occasions when patients really are unable to swallow tablets. Diazepam is an excellent drug for short-term acute anxiety problems but its long-term use is complicated by a high addiction rating and so it is generally contra-indicated for such use.

Midazolam

Midazolam is a water-soluble and fat-soluble benzodiazepine with a much shorter half-life than diazepam. It is prepared in injectable form and is the most commonly used intravenous sedative. It has also been used, however, in clinical trials using the solution as nasal drops, particularly for sedation in children. The results were encouraging but not universally effective. Whether this practice will ever get past experimental usage is difficult to determine but it is probably unlikely unless its success rate can be raised.

Temazepam

Temazepam was until recently one of the most commonly used oral sedatives. It was originally marketed as a hypnotic for inducing sleep but its shorter half-life (circa 4 hours) makes it ideal for use as a sedative. Like diazepam it is highly addictive and in the 1980s it became one of the most commonly abused drugs due to its presentation as 'gelules' and it was made a Category 2 restricted drug in response to this. Despite the problems caused by the drug being abused, temazepam remains one of the most ideal oral sedatives/premedicants due to its shorter half-life and minimal hangover effect. An anxious, otherwise healthy adult of normal weight should be given a dose of 20 mg and the effect assessed after 30 minutes.

The barbiturates

Barbiturates are rarely used nowadays, their use having been almost entirely supplanted by the benzodiazepines and there is now very little indication for their use in pre-operative sedation. Occasionally, the use of pentobarbitone sodium is encountered but it can really only be justified in patients who are hypersensitive to benzodiazepines and this is extremely rare. Drug tolerance and dependence easily occur with all barbiturates although, as mentioned, dependency to the benzodiazepines is also well documented. Additionally, their use in cases of respiratory, renal or hepatic disease should be avoided and the concomitant use of any other central nervous system depressants is contra-indicated. Oral barbiturates should not be given to patients in pain as they may cause confusion and irritability.

Other sedatives

Trimeprazine and promethazine

Trimeprazine and promethazine are effective, H_1-histamine antagonists (antihistamines of the phenothiazine group) and trimeprazine has been found particularly suitable for sedation in children. It is available in tablet or syrup form and has a reasonable anti-emetic action. It should be given in doses of about 2 mg/kg of body weight initially, as higher doses may produce sleep. If the effect is inadequate at this level an increase of 50% of the initial dose should be given. Trimeprazine is available in two concentrations (Vallergan®, Vallergan Forte®) to avoid the need to give large volumes of syrup to bigger children (Figure 7.1). Trimeprazine will often overcome the irrational fear found in

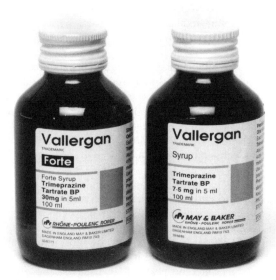

Figure 7.1 Trimeprazine and trimeprazine forte containing 7.5 mg/5 ml and 30 mg/5 ml respectively.

younger children, which is often resistant to small doses of diazepam or temazepam. This is, therefore, particularly useful for out-patient sedation but in hospital where patients can be observed, higher doses of temazepam are usually preferred (also in the hospital situation the phenothiazines may be given in higher doses). The side effects of the phenothiazines include persistent drowsiness, disturbing dreams (or other psychosomatic effects), nasal stuffiness and headaches. Occasional skin rashes and respiratory depression have also been reported.

Promethazine hydrochloride has also been used in the sedation of children, but its use as a sole agent in sedation is generally less satisfactory than that of trimeprazine. Doses of 5 mg to 25 mg can be given orally from the age of 6 months to 10 years on a dose/weight related ratio. Occasionally promethazine has reversed effects producing restlessness, irritability and hallucinations. Fortunately, this is extremely rare at the recommended doses.

The phenothiazines are a useful group of drugs which have an excellent sedative action. This can be employed to great advantage in young children where in particular, trimeprazine is extremely effective in calming an anxious, distraught child.

Triclofos
This is another useful hypnosedative in a non-barbiturate group. It is derived from an old hypnotic known as chloral hydrate. Unlike the latter which tastes foul, however, it is virtually tasteless and is, therefore, useful in very young children. It derives its effect in the same way as chloral hydrate as a result of hydrolysis within the body, when it breaks down into trichloroethanol. It is this metabolite which produces the hypnotic/sedative effects. In addition, it is further metabolized and excreted relatively quickly, this giving a relatively short half-life and infrequent 'hangovers'. It has little if any tendency to cause respiratory

depression and is therefore useful in patients where it is mandatory to avoid this. For children over 1 year of age, a dose of 250 mg or less may be sufficient to produce sleep but doses up to 500 mg may prove necessary in older children. Above the age of 6 years, this may be increased to 1g in the severely anxious, but such high doses occasionally result in non-disturbable sleep. Even so the safety margin is very wide and cardiac and respiratory depression rarely occur.

Triclofos is potentiated in the presence of alcohol, barbiturates, CNS depressants and certain other sedatives and tranquillizers. It may also increase the potency of the coumarin-type anticoagulants and for this reason it should be avoided as a sedative in patients who are receiving this group of drugs.

Side effects may include dizziness, headache and gastro-intestinal upsets but the drug is relatively free of serious complications. It is contra-indicated in patients with severe renal, hepatic or cardiac impairment. Triclofos is no longer a commonly used drug, particularly in out-patients but this is more due to the advent of the new hypnosedatives, rather than to its lack of efficiency which is basically quite satisfactory.

The opiates (narcotics)

For the sake of completeness it is important to consider these naturally-occurring substances which are frequently used in hospital practice but have no place in the dental surgery. The original opiates were naturally-occurring alkaloids of opium, an extract of the wild poppy seed. Similar powerful synthetic forms are available, each with its own individual variations in properties. In general terms each drug will to a greater or lesser extent relieve pain, induce sedation and produce a combination of stimulatory and depressant actions in the central nervous system. All opiates demonstrate a fairly powerful synergy with the benzodiazepines and so their use should be restricted to hospital practice with a second person administering the sedation. The use of a combined opiate/benzodiazepine technique which gained some popularity in the last decade cannot be recommended in any way as a safe procedure for the operator/sedationist and it is questionable if it should ever be used in an out-patient situation.

All opiates may cause quite severe side effects due to their basic pharmaco-kinetic action (e.g. depression of the cough and laryngeal reflexes) and great care should be taken in administering them. It is also important to be aware of the addictive nature of the opiates, which is both physical and psychological. There is some evidence that the risk of addiction is at its lowest when these drugs are administered intramuscularly.

Premedication is seldom necessary for the dental out-patient but, when it is required, there is no place for the opiates. For in-patient procedures, however, they are in common usage, particularly fentanyl, morphine, pethidine and papaveretum (see below). Their main advantage is that their action can be reversed in an emergency with the use of naloxone (Figure 7.2). The main criticism is that it is illogical to give powerful analgesics to patients with minimal or no pain and there is little evidence to suggest they are any more effective as analgesics than the non-steroidal anti-inflammatory medications such as ibuprofen. Despite this they retain their popularity with a large number of anaesthetists.

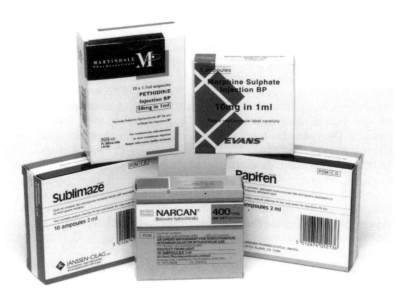

Figure 7.2 Various opiates with naloxone which is capable of reversing their action in an emergency. Opiates have a symbiotic effect with the benzodiazepines and the combination is not suitable for out-patient conscious sedation.

Fentanyl

Fentanyl is a synthetic opiate which is chemically similar to pethidine but has a much higher potency by a factor of 600–700. It is available in slightly differing forms and is relatively short-acting (20–40 minutes maximum). The use of fentanyl in combination with benzodiazepines produces profound sedation, often with severe respiratory depression and so this technique should be regarded as one of anaesthesia rather than sedation. Like most of the opiates fentanyl can be reversed by the administration of naloxone; even so its use should be reserved for occasions when the operator is not the person administering the sedation. A similar but less potent variant known as alfentanil is also available.

Morphine

In its basic form it occurs as a natural alkaloid but is commercially available as the hydrochloride or sulphate. It is a powerful depressant of the cough reflex, pain response and respiratory frequency. It stimulates the vomiting reflex and the action of the pupillary muscles of the eye and suppresses the action of the intestinal muscles.

However, the production of euphoric feelings still make morphine a popular premedicant when used in conjunction with an anti-emetic. A dose of 5–20 mg may be given but the standard dose for a healthy adult is 10 mg. By tradition, this dose given to a healthy adult has been used as a basis for comparison with other analgesics.

Papaveretum

Papaveretum is less powerful in its effects than morphine and is also said to have fewer side effects. It does certainly appear to produce less nausea but it is difficult to assess whether this is because relatively smaller doses are given (normally 10–20 mg for adults). The actual mixture of papaveretum has an equivalent morphine content of half its actual weight. As with morphine it is usually given in conjunction with an anti-emetic.

Pethidine
Pethidine is a less powerful analgesic than fentanyl, morphine or papaveretum (morphine is about ten times more effective). It is one of the synthetic narcotics and, possibly because of its lower potency, has fewer side effects than fentanyl, morphine or papaveretum. A dose of between 25 and 100 mg is given but an adjunct, usually of the phenothiazine group, is commonly administered to ensure adequate sedation without nausea.

All the narcotics rely on the liver and kidneys for their breakdown and excretion so should not be administered to patients with known hepatic or renal disease. It is recommended that pethidine (and probably all the natural opiates) should be avoided in patients who are taking monoamine oxidase inhibitors, as indirect drug interactions can occur. The opiates should also be avoided in many of the diseases mentioned in Chapter 1.

Clinical use of the hypnosedatives

It is probably true to say that virtually every drug in this category has been tried at some time as a sedation agent or to premedicate patients. The effects of individual drugs vary but, as in sedation itself, the benzodiazepines enjoy prime position in terms of popular usage. These drugs have been used orally and despite the theoretical problems which may arise from needing a drink to swallow the capsule, this has not been a clinical problem.

Diazepam remains a dependable oral sedative which has excellent soporific effects but given orally it produces minimal amnesia. It can be given by intramuscular injection if required but given intramuscularly its action is less consistent and if parenteral use is required, immediate pre-operative intravenous injection is probably preferable. This is a particularly useful technique when anaesthesia with ketamine is contemplated, as it will usually eliminate the vestibular and visual disturbances which commonly occur postoperatively.

The use of phenothiazines (which are now usually regarded as minor tranquillizers) in premedication is becoming less common. They are useful anti-emetics and are sometimes used in the preparation of patients with fractured jaws who are going to have their jaws fixed in the closed position with either intra-oral or extra-oral fixation. It is more usual nowadays to give such drugs postoperatively and give drugs such as droperidol during an anaesthetic which are themselves anti-emetic. It should be noted that when using in-patient general anaesthesia, some anaesthetists still prefer the 'grand slam', giving a narcotic analgesic, an antihistamine and an anti-sialogogue.

The concept of premedication

Although the purpose of premedication is to produce a sedated patient, it may be defined as the administration of a drug or drugs before either sedation (or anaesthetic) which assists in facilitating both the operation and the sedation (or anaesthetic) and recovery. Premedication is, therefore, a clinical concept and the drugs used to produce the sedative element are largely those of oral sedation (see above). However, premedication can also be used on occasion for other reasons such as reducing salivary and bronchial secretions, lessening the response to painful stimuli and reducing the risk of vomiting. Of the different types of drugs available to produce sedation are the various categories of drugs that have been mentioned earlier.

It should be mentioned that the term 'narcotic' is a pharmacological term (meaning sleep-producing) whilst hypnosedative and tranquillizer are actually clinical terms. The distinguishing of these different groups is, therefore, not easy since there is considerable overlap between the clinical and pharmacological properties.

In terms of the other effects required with premedication, however, it is easier to distinguish the anti-emetics, the anti-sialogogues and the analgesics although there is a degree of functional overlap with these agents which are outlined below:

The anti-emetics

The use of anti-emetics should always be considered if there is any likelihood that opiates are to be administered or in patients with a history of anxiety-induced vomiting. Anxious patients frequently feel nauseous, many have marked retching reflexes and those with severe anxiety do occasionally vomit. In these situations anti-emetics are useful in suppressing the vomiting reflex and often have the added benefit of providing some supplementary sedation. The most common anti-emetics are found in the phenothiazine group of drugs with perphenazine, perchlorperazine and metoclopramide probably being the most commonly used. Many others are available and some are even purchasable without prescription as motion sickness relievers. The antihistamines have also occasionally been given to reduce nausea but their effect is less well documented and certainly less profound than the phenothiazines. Ultra-potent anti-emetics such as odansetron should rarely be required but can be administered to patients suffering with intractable vomiting.

The anti-sialogogues

An anti-sialogogue is a drug which suppresses secretions of the salivary glands. The most common way of achieving this is to prevent the secretomotor action of acetylcholine. Pharmacologically similar drugs, atropine, hyoscine and glyco-pyrrolate are used virtually exclusively in this area.

The first two are natural alkaloids not totally dissimilar from cocaine in their chemical formula. Despite their similarities in structure and in reducing secreto-motor activity they do have some fundamentally different effects on the central nervous system. In particular, the standard dose for a healthy adult of 0.6 mg of atropine (usually given intramuscularly) will cause an initial bradycardia of very short duration, followed by a more prolonged tachycardia. For some reason intravenous injection less commonly results in the initial bradycardia. The anti-sialogogue effect of atropine is said by some to be less than that of hyoscine, but research has shown the difference to be insignificant. All the anti-sialogogues have the advantage of being available as oral preparations.

The cardiovascular effects of glycopyrrolate (and hyoscine) are far less marked than those of atropine and if a slight tachycardia occurs it seldom reaches a rate where arrhythmias may result (which is the case with atropine). Hyoscine has the added advantage of being a reasonably effective anti-emetic; it does not produce the same cardiac effects and does not cause any degree of tachycardia. Hyoscine has another advantage over atropine and glycopyrrolate in that it causes 'twilight sleep' when used in association with the narcotic analgesics. This results in a fairly profound sedation and is often followed by a reasonable degree of analgesia. It is not a technique for the single administrator/operator, however.

The analgesics

Analgesia may be given as part of premedication for two reasons. Initially it may provide a raised pain threshold for painful stimuli such as local injections and subsequently it may provide postoperative pain relief. There is good evidence that patients perceive lower levels of pain if it is suppressed before it becomes significantly established and there are now large numbers of well-controlled clinical trials showing the benefit of many analgesics.

With little doubt the most effective of these are the non-steroidal anti-inflammatory group of drugs (NSAIDs) of which the best-known and probably the one with least side effects is ibuprofen. However, there are many different agents available in a variety of forms and the use of per rectal diclofenac (Voltarol®) is currently popular. However, in general dental practice extreme caution should be employed before any decision is made to administer drugs via the rectum as, without explicit consent, a practitioner would be guilty of assault and battery. More potent NSAIDs (e.g. Ketorolac®; ketoprofen) have also been developed but these do seem to be associated with a higher incidence of side effects and their routine use is probably not indicated.

The use of paracetamol-based drugs is the next most effective form of oral analgesia. These are available in many forms, often with the addition of codeine at varying levels. There is little scientific evidence to show that the codeine has any beneficial effect, particularly at the lower levels when the dose is almost certainly subtherapeutic. Thus, paracetamol-based preparations with codeine 8 mg added are unlikely to be any more effective than the paracetamol 500 mg alone. There is some suggestion that once the codeine dose increases to 30 mg in 500 mg, the benefit has been shown to be clinically detectable although it is only marginally significant.

Finally, mention should be made again of the opiates. There is little evidence to suggest that opiates are any more effective than NSAIDs in relieving the pain of acute inflammation but their use in the treatment of severe pain remains popular with many anaesthetists. It is mandatory to remember the synergistic nature of the benzodiazepine/opiate combination and their use in out-patient situations cannot be recommended.

Adequate pain relief should always be given a high priority in the management of any patient and this has frequently not been given enough consideration. It is not acceptable to discharge patients who may experience severe postoperative pain without checking and providing sufficient analgesia. As mentioned earlier, pain relief is most effective if it is tackled before it is well established and this explains the rationale behind the use of analgesics in premedication. However, postoperative pain management remains the responsibility of the surgeon and should always be given adequate attention.

Other drugs

In conclusion, it should be mentioned that other drugs may need to be administered during premedication. Included in this would be antibiotics to cover patients with cardiac defects and steroids for those requiring cover due to taking steroid medication or because they suffer from adrenal insufficiency. These drugs do not fit the concept or definition of premedication but, none the less, can frequently be given simultaneously. It is clearly important that the dental surgeon considers all the agents which may require administration and that they are given at the appropriate time using the best means of access.

References and further reading

Healy, T.E.J. and Cohen, P.J. (eds) (1995). *Wylie and Churchill-Davidson's A Practice of Anaesthesia*. London: Arnold.

Hill, C.M. and Morris, P.J. (1991). *General Anaesthesia and Sedation in Dentistry*, 2nd edn. London: Wright.

Whitwam, J.G. (ed.) (1994). *Day-case Anaesthesia and Sedation*. London: Blackwell.

8

Complications and emergencies

Introduction

Sedation in dentistry has a very good safety record. If intravenous, inhalational or oral sedation is administered correctly to carefully selected patients by trained dental surgeons with appropriate facilities and support, then the incidence of untoward problems should be very low. However, complications can and do occur and it is essential that all dental surgeons practising sedation should be trained in the management of sedation-related complications and medical emergencies. Unfortunately, most problems arise from irresponsibility on the part of the dental surgeon. It is not usually the drugs or techniques used in sedation which are at fault but the clinician that administers them.

By definition, a true emergency is one which occurs without warning and which could not reasonably have been foreseen. Medical emergencies can affect anyone, at any time, irrespective of whether they are at home, at work, walking down the street or in a dental surgery. Thankfully such emergencies are rare but even so every dental surgeon has the responsibility to be able to manage such problems if they arise. All members of the dental team should be trained and regularly updated in the recognition and management of medical emergencies and in current techniques of basic life support. The dental surgeon practising sedation should also have some knowledge of the methods of advanced life support since these are critically important in the successful resuscitation of a collapsed patient. It is also the responsibility of the dental surgeon to ensure that he has appropriate equipment and drugs available ready for use if an emergency should arise.

Many sedation-related complications are predictable and thus emergencies should be avoidable by good planning and skilful technique. The need for careful and thorough pre-sedation patient assessment cannot be over-emphasized. The fitness of each patient to undergo treatment under sedation, and thus the risk which sedation presents to the patient, must be individually assessed. If any aspect of the medical history suggests a potential problem then expert advice should be sought, either from the patient's medical practitioner or by referral to a hospital specialist. Dental treatment requiring sedation is never so urgent as to put the patient's life at risk from inadequate assessment and planning.

Every dental surgeon undertaking sedation must ensure that he is suitably qualified and experienced. Postgraduate training in sedation is mandatory, with a minimum requirement of attendance at a postgraduate course. The course should not only cover the theoretical and practical aspects of conscious sedation but must also provide hands-on supervised clinical experience. The dental surgeon should appreciate the need for good teamwork between himself/herself, the dental nurse and other members of the practice staff. Dental nurses should receive individual sedation training so that they can assist in the care of patients undergoing sedation and be able to help in the management of emergencies. The dental surgeon must also ensure that his/her practice has appropriate facilities to undertake sedation and to deal with any emergency that may arise.

Although all dental practices should be equally prepared for the management of an emergency, those that provide sedation have an extra duty of care because of the inherent additional risks of treating patients under sedation. Adherence to the principles of good sedation practice should minimize the incidence of untoward problems. However, despite careful preparation and technique, complications and emergencies can still arise. This chapter will discuss the emergency equipment and drugs required when practising sedation, the aetiology, clinical features and management of specific sedation-related problems and medical emergencies and the prevention and treatment of local complications.

Emergency equipment and drugs

In the dental surgery there is a limit to the emergency facilities which can and should be provided. Various bodies have attempted to provide exhaustive lists of emergency equipment and drugs that should be kept in dental practices. Many of the recommendations include drugs which a dental surgeon would never be expected to use. A good rule of thumb is that the dental surgery should stock equipment and drugs which are essential to manage the more common medical emergencies and to provide a high standard of basic life support. The dental surgeon should understand the effects of the various drugs and be competent to use all of the items stocked. At the current time, equipment and drugs for advanced life support are only mandatory in practices providing general anaesthesia, which is outside the remit of this book.

Emergency equipment

Every practice undertaking sedation should stock a ventilating device for administering oxygen under intermittent positive pressure. This is used to support ventilation in a patient who becomes significantly hypnoeic, apnoeic or has a respiratory arrest. The classic example is the 'Ambu-bag' which consists of a self-inflating bag, with an oxygen attachment, one-way valve and face mask (Figure 8.1). When attached to an oxygen supply this bag will deliver approximately 40% oxygen in air. A higher percentage of oxygen, up to 80%, can be administered by attaching an oxygen reservoir bag to the main self-inflating bag. The Ambu-bag requires two people to operate it efficiently, one to hold the mask on the face to maintain a good seal and to support the airway, the other to squeeze the bag and ventilate the patient. It is possible to use the Ambu-bag single-handedly but it can be difficult to perform these tasks simultaneously.

Another example of an intermittent positive-pressure device is the simple pocket-mask with an oxygen attachment (Figure 8.2). This is easier to use by a

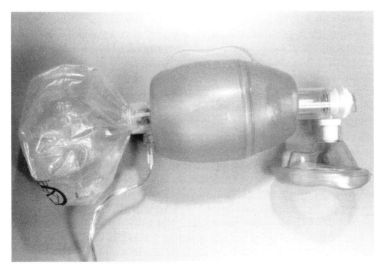

Figure 8.1 Self-inflating positive-pressure ventilation bag, with reservoir and oxygen attachment (Ambu bag).

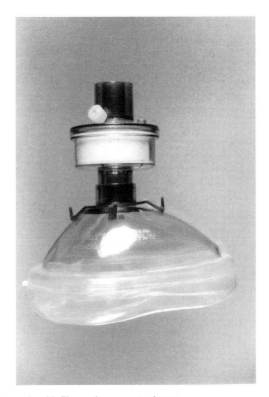

Figure 8.2 Pocket-mask, with filter and oxygen attachment.

single person than the Ambu-bag because all the manual effort is aimed at holding the mask in position and maintaining the airway. Ventilation is achieved by the practitioner actually breathing into the mask. The percentage of oxygen delivered is less than that achieved with an Ambu-bag, but the device is easier to operate and may be more efficient than an improperly used Ambu-bag.

The dental practice must have a selection of Guedel oral airways (Figure 8.3). These are used to maintain a patent airway in an unconscious patient. The commonest cause of airway obstruction in the unconscious patient is caused by the tongue falling back onto the anterior wall of the pharynx. This problem can usually be relieved by placing the patient in the lateral recovery position or by pulling the mandible forwards using the chin lift or jaw thrust. A simple means of assisting airway maintenance is to insert a Guedel oral airway. This sits over the back of the tongue, preventing it falling posteriorly into the pharynx. Air can then pass freely in and out via the hollow airway lumen. The oral airway requires careful insertion to ensure that the tongue is not pushed backwards upon insertion. For this reason it is inserted upside down as far as the back of the hard palate (Figure 8.4), when it is turned over into the correct orientation (Figure 8.5). The Guedel airway can only be used in an unconscious patient. It will be forcefully ejected once the patient regains consciousness and the pharyngeal reflexes return.

Portable suction equipment (preferably totally independent of the main suction supply) should always be available (Figure 8.6). Good suction is essential when undertaking sedation but an emergency back-up system should always be available. Although the laryngeal reflexes in a sedated patient are usually intact they do have a reduced gag reflex and less ability to remove vomit or foreign bodies from the mouth. The suction apparatus should be portable so that it can be used in the recovery area or any other part of the dental practice. It should also be independent of the power supply so it will still function if there is a power failure. Manual suction devices are available which do not require a power source.

The most important piece of emergency equipment (or drugs) is an independent

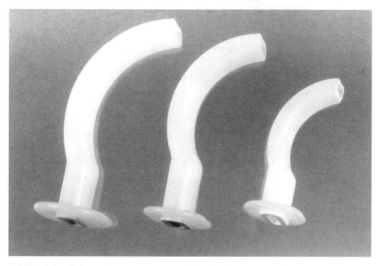

Figure 8.3 Guedel oral airways.

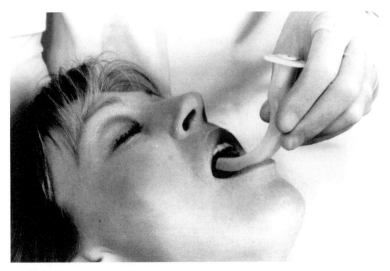

Figure 8.4 Oral airway is initially inserted upside down.

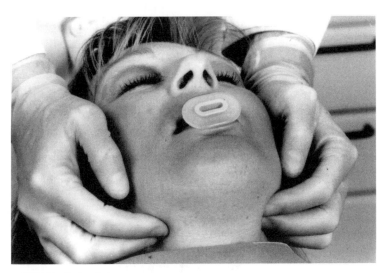

Figure 8.5 Fully sited oral airway.

oxygen supply (Figure 8.7). A full oxygen cylinder, size D (340 litres) or size E (680 litres), which is independent of any routine oxygen supply should be available for an emergency. The cylinder must have a reducing valve, key, flow meter, tubing and suitable connectors. It must be readily attachable to a face mask, nasal cannula, Ambu-bag or pocket-mask. It is essential that the level of oxygen in the cylinder is checked before the start of a sedation session and the cylinder should be turned on ready for immediate use if necessary. Cylinders should be stored on a portable trolley so that they can be used anywhere in the practice.

A range of disposable syringes (5 ml and 2 ml) and needles (23 g) should be available to administer parenteral drugs in an emergency. A selection of butter-

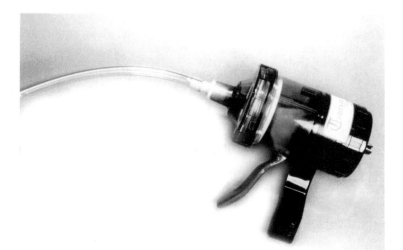

Figure 8.6 Portable mechanical suction device.

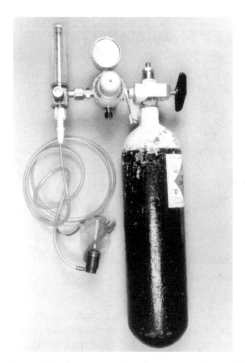

Figure 8.7 Oxygen cylinder with reducing valve, key, flow meter, tubing and face mask.

fly needles or Teflonated cannulae (20 g) should also be kept in the emergency stock so that additional venous access can be gained should the original sedation cannula become blocked or dislodged.

The final piece of essential emergency equipment is a portable cricothyroidotomy kit (Figure 8.8). This provides the facility to perform a cricothyroidotomy to establish a patent airway if the air passages become completely obstructed. This normally occurs when a foreign body is inhaled and becomes lodged in the larynx. If the obstruction is not expelled conventionally by the patient coughing, by back or abdominal thrusts, the Heimlich manoeuvre should be used (see later). If this still fails to clear the airway the patient will become cyanotic and another airway must be established or the patient will suffer a cardiorespiratory arrest.

The cricothyroidotomy kit contains all the equipment required to make an orifice in the cricothyroid membrane and to establish a temporary alternative airway. The neck should be extended and the trachea punctured between the cricoid and thyroid cartilages, just below the Adam's apple (Figure 8.9).

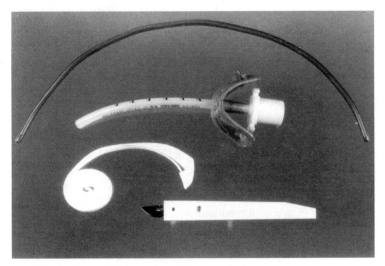

Figure 8.8 Cricothyoidotomy kit containing a sheathed scalpel, a size 4 portex tracheostomy airway, inserting device and securing tape.

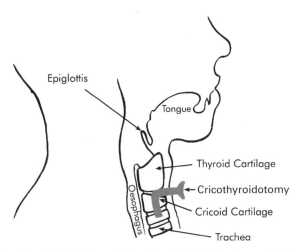

Epiglottis

Tongue

Thyroid Cartilage

Cricothyroidotomy

Cricoid Cartilage

Oesophagus

Trachea

Figure 8.9 Penetration of the skin should be made just below the Adam's apple, see also Figure 8.14.

Emergency drugs

Certain emergency drugs should always be stocked in a practice undertaking sedation. It is essential that the dental surgeon understands the indication for each drug and how it is administered. There is little point in stocking a drug if it cannot be used appropriately.

The most important 'drug' for any dental practice to stock is oxygen. This is the first and, in many cases, the only substance which is required in an emergency situation. It is of particular importance in sedation because almost all sedation agents produce some degree of respiratory depression. The normal concentration of oxygen in the air is 21%. By administering 100% oxygen from a cylinder, via a nasal cannula or face mask, the inspired percentage of oxygen can be significantly increased. This will help to compensate for the slight desaturation that can occur as a result of mild respiratory depression. The administration of 100% oxygen is also an essential first step in the management of nearly all medical emergencies.

Adrenaline at a concentration of 1 mg/1 ml (1 in 1000 dilution) is required for the treatment of anaphylaxis. Adrenaline is administered either intramuscularly or subcutaneously. It should **never** be delivered via the intravenous route in general dental practice although it can be used in this way, usually in a more dilute form, in some hospital situations. Adrenaline may also be required for the treatment of severe asthmatic bronchospasm.

Hydrocortisone hemisuccinate (100 mg/2 ml) should be stocked for the management of an adrenal crisis, anaphylaxis and severe asthma. It is presented as an anhydrous hydrocortisone powder and a separate ampoule of water. The two are mixed together immediately before administration. Hydrocortisone can be delivered intramuscularly, subcutaneously or intravenously. It is probably best administered via the intravenous route when the 100 mg hydrocortisone powder should be diluted into 10 ml of water and given relatively slowly.

Chlorpheniramine maleate (10 mg/1 ml) is an antihistamine which should be available for the management of minor allergic reactions. It is presented in solution and is administered intramuscularly or intravenously. Antihistamines have little place in the immediate management of anaphylaxis since it is not principally histamine mediated but they are still recommended in a supportive role.

Glucose or dextrose tablets or gel should be available for use in the early stages of a hypoglycaemic attack in a diabetic patient. A conscious patient should be given tablets to suck or the gel can be smoothed onto the oral mucosa. Alternatively, a glucose-based drink can be given. However, if the patient's condition is deteriorating there should be no hesitation about giving intravenous glucose or parenteral glucagon (see below).

Glucagon (1 mg) is required if the hypoglycaemic patient loses consciousness. It is administered intramuscularly. Sterile glucose or dextrose (50 ml of a 50% solution) which is delivered intravenously should also be available. This is more rapidly acting than glucagon but its high viscosity can make it difficult to administer through the narrow bore cannulae used to administer sedation drugs. A 25% dilution is also available and rather more easy to administer.

Glyceryl trinitrate tablets (0.5 mg) or glyceryl trinitrate spray (0.4 mg/dose) is required for the management of angina. Both tablets and spray are administered sublingually to maximize the rate of absorption.

Aspirin tablets (300 mg) should be stocked for use in the event of a myocardial infarction. Aspirin reduces platelet adhesiveness and is used to reduce the morbidity of myocardial infarction. There is good evidence that early administration improves morbidity and reduces mortality after myocardial infarction.

A salbutamol inhaler (0.1 mg/dose) or a salbutamol nebulizer with nebules (2.5 mg) should be available for the management of an acute asthma attack. Very severe asthma attacks may require treatment with adrenaline but this should only be administered once an ECG has been placed so that its effects on the heart can be carefully observed. This technique should be reserved for the hospital environment and is not appropriate for use in general dental practice.

Diazepam emulsion (10 mg/2 ml) is recommended for the treatment of *status epilepticus*. Although this should be stocked for use in an emergency, any patient who has already received midazolam sedation can be given further midazolam for the treatment of a fit, care being taken not to over-dose the patient. Both benzodiazepines have similar anticonvulsant properties.

All of the above emergency drugs should be available in a dental practice, irrespective of whether sedation is being provided or not. The only additional emergency drug which must be stocked where sedation is being practised is the benzodiazepine antagonist, flumazenil (500 mg/5 ml). Alongside oxygen, this is probably the most useful drug for dealing with emergencies arising as a result of over-sedation. However, it does not obviate the need for instituting basic life support procedures at the first sign of any untoward problem.

Other drugs have been recommended for inclusion in the emergency stock. Most other emergency drugs are only indicated for advanced life support and their usefulness requires individual assessment. Opiates are not recommended for simple sedation but if they are being used for any reason it is essential that the antagonist, naloxone, is stocked with the emergency drugs. A dental surgeon undertaking simple conscious sedation with nitrous oxide or the benzodiazepines would not be expected to stock or use these additional drugs unless he/she were familiar with the detailed techniques of advanced life support.

Since there is good evidence that early defibrillation is the key to successful resuscitation after cardiac arrest, it is likely that there will be a growing demand for sedationists and dentists to be trained in advanced life support. Although this may seem a distant prospect, with the advent of technologically competent defibrillators (Figure 8.10) which will literally talk someone through the emergency procedure, the likelihood of it becoming more accepted is ever increasing.

Sedation-related emergencies

The treatment of patients under sedation carries a number of inherent potential risks. Whilst it is essential to be prepared for an emergency it is better to prevent one occurring by maintaining a high state of awareness. The key to successful management of emergencies is early identification and intervention. When a patient is being treated under sedation the dental surgeon and dental nurse should be continuously aware of the patency of the airway, rate and depth of breathing, heart rate, arterial oxygen saturation, skin colour and level of consciousness. Careful clinical monitoring, supplemented with pulse oximetry, is

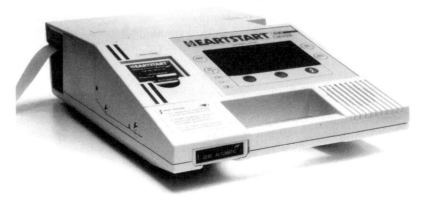

Figure 8.10 The 'intelligent' defibrillator. The machine will only allow a discharge of current once it has diagnosed defibrillation. In addition it talks (literally) to the clinician with instructions on what to do.

mandatory. At the first sign of any untoward problem dental treatment should immediately be terminated and full attention must be paid to the patient's clinical status.

Any significant alteration of clinical signs, such as a reduction in respiration rate or pulse rate, should prompt the dental surgeon to take immediate action. For example if a patient becomes pale and nauseous during the induction of sedation this may indicate an impending vasovagal attack. Unless the patient is rapidly laid supine they will lose consciousness. This is not the effect of the sedation drug (although it may be compounded by it) but is a simple faint.

Careful monitoring of the patient's clinical status will alert the dental surgeon to the early signs of an untoward problem. Failing to observe or ignoring the signs of impending problems and delaying management is negligent on the part of the practitioner and may put the patient at serious risk.

The pulse oximeter can be very useful in providing an early warning of impending problems developing. For example a drop in oxygen saturation will normally be identified by the oximeter long before any clinical signs of de-saturation appear. If the dental surgeon intervenes immediately then the problem can be corrected using simple measures. Slight oxygen de-saturation can be reversed by asking the patient to breathe deeply or by the administration of nasal oxygen. However, if the dental surgeon fails to intervene early the problem can become difficult to manage and may even become life threatening.

A number of complications and emergencies relate specifically to sedation. It is worthwhile considering the features and management of sedation-related problems in comparison with standard medical emergencies. The dental surgeon practising sedation must be able to distinguish between sedation-related emergencies and medical emergencies occurring in the sedated patient.

Anxiety-related problems

Patients undergoing sedation are often acutely anxious and very prone to having a vasovagal attack (faint). This usually occurs during cannulation or in the early stages of sedative drug administration. It can be largely averted by laying the patient supine prior to commencing the procedure. However, if a patient does become pale, clammy and nauseous then the most likely cause is vasovagal syncope. The patient should immediately be laid flat with the legs raised and any drug administration stopped (Figure 8.11). If the patient becomes unconscious the airway should be maintained and oxygen administered via a face mask. Consciousness should be rapidly regained, although the patient may be drowsy due to the effect of any sedation agent administered prior to the faint. Severe faints, i.e. those where consciousness is lost, can also result in minor epileptiform activity. This should not be confused with an epileptic attack which is progressive unlike a faint, when the shaking stops rapidly once the blood circulation to the brain has been re-established.

Severe anxiety can also precipitate an acute exacerbation of a pre-existing medical condition, such as angina, asthma or epilepsy. Even patients with apparently well-controlled medical conditions can deteriorate when presented with a situation which increases anxiety. Such acute medical problems may present at any stage during the sedation appointment and should be treated using the standard protocols which are discussed later in this chapter. For most cases of pre-existing disease, appropriate precautions should have been taken to minimize the chance of precipitating an acute exacerbation. However, it is still essential to have all equipment and drugs that might be required to manage a potential emergency readily available at the chair-side.

Respiratory depression

The most likely complication of benzodiazepine sedation is respiratory depression. This is known to occur with all benzodiazepines but it is not usually of any

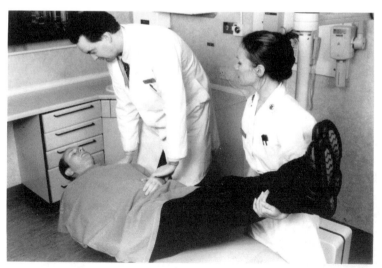

Figure 8.11 A patient who has a vasovagal attack should be laid supine with the legs raised to encourage venous return to the heart. They should be closely monitored until consciousness is regained.

clinical significance and the arterial blood remains well saturated. However, excessively rapid intravenous administration, benzodiazepine over-dosage or adverse drug interaction can have a significant effect on the respiratory system. In addition, the very young and very old are particularly sensitive to the respiratory depressant effects of intravenous sedative agents. Careful patient selection, slow titration of the sedation agent and continuous clinical and electromechanical monitoring will minimize the risk. If there is any evidence of respiratory compromise this should be corrected immediately by maintaining the airway, administering oxygen and if necessary by providing assisted positive-pressure ventilation (Figure 8.12). If the oxygen saturation falls and cannot be restored with simple measures then the respiratory depressant effects of the sedation should be reversed by administering 200–500 μg of flumazenil. Respiratory depression was much more common when a two-drug approach was used (e.g. a benzodiazepine and an opiate) and should rarely be encountered nowadays.

Airway obstruction

Airway obstruction by aspiration of a foreign body is a potential hazard of treating patients under sedation. Sedation causes some reduction in the gag reflex and if a tooth, a piece of amalgam or a reamer is dropped to the back of the mouth the patient may find it difficult to expel the foreign body. Good airway protection using a butterfly sponge or rubber dam and high volume suction should avoid the occurrence of this problem. If a foreign body does fall into the larynx and the patient starts to choke they should be leant forward, or turned into the prone position, and encouraged to cough. The dental surgeon should assist by firmly slapping the patient's back just between the scapulae. If this does not dislodge the foreign body the dental surgeon or

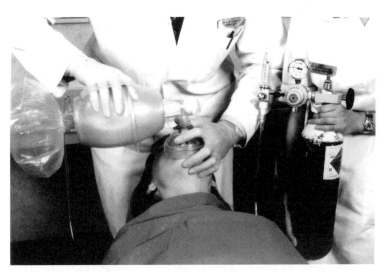

Figure 8.12 Positive-pressure ventilation should be commenced immediately if a patient becomes apnoeic or significantly hypnoeic.

his assistant should perform the Heimlich manoeuvre (Figure 8.13). Positioning oneself behind the patient the dental surgeon should clasp his/her hands firmly around the patient's waist. Firm pressure applied to the abdomen just below the xiphisternum will force the diaphragm up and the expired air should expel the foreign body. If it is not possible to stand the patient up they should be placed on their side with the head as low down as possible. The dental surgeon may then stand in front of the patient and give abdominal thrusts, again from just below the xiphisternum, to try and dislodge the foreign body.

Where the foreign body cannot be expelled and there is airway obstruction with little or no air entry, the only option is to perform a cricothyroidotomy (Figure 8.14). The head is extended by placing a bag of saline underneath the neck. The cricoid and thyroid cartilages are palpated and the depression between the two, the cricothyroid membrane, is located. A small, vertical incision is made through the skin and cricothyroid membrane. The cricothyroid cannula is inserted through the orifice created and into the trachea. A connector is attached to the cannula and oxygen is administered at the highest flow rate possible. The cannula is secured in place with tape passed around the neck. The cannula will allow enough air entry until expert assistance arrives and can be life-saving.

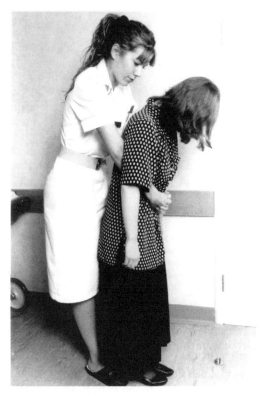

Figure 8.13 The Heimlich manoeuvre.

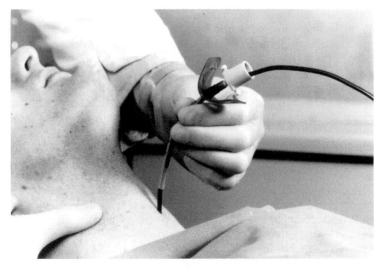

Figure 8.14 Cricothyroidotomy. The neck is extended and a small vertical incision is made through the skin and the cricothyroid membrane in the midline of the neck. The cricothyroid airway is inserted into the trachea over a rigid introducer. Oxygen is then administered at the maximum flow rate.

Drug interactions

The use of the intravenous route of sedation drug administration may result in more rapid and severe drug reactions and interactions. Anaphylaxis, drug idiosyncrasy and drug interactions can all occur with intravenous sedation. An awareness of any previous reaction to a drug and slow incremental administration of the sedation agent with cessation of administration should any untoward problems occur, will minimize the onset and severity of drug complications.

Drug interactions vary in severity and are more difficult to manage. At the first sign of any untoward reaction the administration of the sedation agent should be stopped and the patient's clinical status should be monitored. Basic life support measures should be initiated if necessary and expert assistance summoned. A true anaphylactic reaction should be treated using the standard protocol described in the next section.

Loss of consciousness

By definition, patients undergoing conscious sedation should never lose consciousness. However, unconsciousness does sometimes occur as a direct result of sedation. It usually results from the administration of an excessive dose of sedation agent, drug idiosyncrasy or drug interaction. It may also be caused by an untoward medical emergency, totally unconnected to the sedation, such as cardiac arrest, epileptic attack, diabetic coma, adrenal crisis or stroke. Sedation-related causes of unconsciousness can be avoided by obtaining a detailed drug history and by slow and careful titration of the sedation agent related to the patient's response. If the patient shows signs of over-sedation and becomes unresponsive to command then oxygen should be administered.

If the oxygen saturation cannot be maintained at a satisfactory level the sedation should be reversed by administering flumazenil. No operative treatment should be undertaken until the patient returns to an acceptable level of sedation.

Patients who become unconscious should be placed on their side and the airway should be maintained. Assistance must be immediately summoned and the patient monitored closely for signs of cardiorespiratory compromise. If the loss of consciousness is the result of over-sedation, the patient should regain consciousness within 2–3 minutes of receiving the reversal agent. If they still remain unconscious then a medical cause should be suspected, identified and managed using standard protocols. A dental surgeon providing a sedation service should be competent to undertake the immediate management of sedation-related emergencies. However, he/she should not hesitate to call the emergency services if there is any concern about a patient's clinical status.

Medical emergencies

Medical emergencies are largely unpredictable and can occur in any patients, whether they are undergoing sedation or not. It requires greater vigilance to identify medical emergencies which occur during sedation and it can be difficult to distinguish them from specific sedation-related complications. Nevertheless, the clinical features and management of specific medical emergencies is the same irrespective of whether they occur in a sedated or a fully conscious patient. Every dental surgeon should be able to recognize and manage a medical emergency; for the dental sedationist there is an extra duty of care.

Cardiac arrest

The most serious medical emergency is a cardiac arrest. This can occur for a variety of reasons including as a result of hypoxia, myocardial infarction, anaphylaxis or severe hypotension. Any state which causes respiratory obstruction or apnoea will lead to respiratory arrest and ultimately, if not treated, cardiac arrest.

The cardinal signs of cardiac arrest are unconsciousness and no central pulse. The diagnosis should be made on the basis of the careful observation of these two signs alone and management should be immediate. It must not be delayed whilst waiting for the late signs of cardiac arrest which include cyanosis, no blood pressure and pupil dilatation.

The basic protocol for managing a cardiac arrest or any medical emergency, can be easily remembered as follows:

A = Assess and Airway—assess responsiveness, establish and maintain the airway.

B = Breathing—check breathing and if necessary provide artificial ventilation.

C = Circulation—check the pulse and if indicated commence cardiac massage.

If a cardiac arrest is suspected, the patient's responsiveness is first assessed by shouting and shaking. If there is no response, assistance should be summoned by shouting for help and telephoning for an emergency ambulance. After checking for any oral obstruction, the patient's airway is then opened by extending the neck and protruding the mandible into a Class III position. This can be achieved either by pulling the anterior mandible forwards and upwards (the chin lift, see Figure 8.15) or by the jaw thrust—pushing forward at both angles of the mandible. The mouth should again be examined for vomit or debris, which can be removed using suction or a finger sweep. The dental surgeon must then check for signs of breathing by listening at the mouth, whilst observing and palpating the chest for movement. If there is no breathing, the dental surgeon should commence artificial respiration. Using a pocket mask or Ambu-bag, attached to the emergency oxygen, two full ventilations should be given (Figure 8.16).

After clearing the airway, checking for breathing and (if necessary) ventilating the patient, a pulse should be sought. Ideally, one should palpate the carotid pulse (which is felt anterior to the sternomastoid muscle) for a maximum of 10 seconds (Figure 8.17). If a pulse is present artificial respiration should be continued with regular checks on the pulse. This sequence is continued until breathing recommences or expert help arrives. If the patient does start breathing he/she should be placed into the lateral recovery position and 100% oxygen administered via a face mask.

If at any stage there is no pulse or it becomes undetectable, full cardiopulmonary resuscitation must be instituted immediately. If for some reason the dentist is alone, two slow ventilations should be given followed by fifteen chest compressions (Figure 8.18). The dental surgeon's hands should be clasped together and positioned over the lower third of the sternum. The chest is compressed to a depth of 4–5 cm at a rate of 100 per minute. The fifteen compressions are followed by two ventilations. This sequence is continued until the pulse is restored or until expert assistance arrives. If the pulse and breathing are restored, which is very unlikely, the patient should be placed in the recovery position and 100% oxygen administered. In practice, a fully trained assistant should always be available and the procedure is slightly different. Five compres-

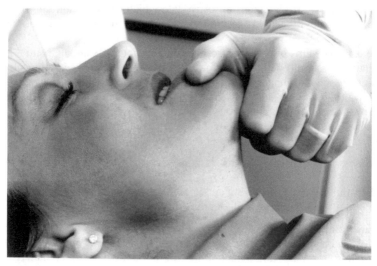

Figure 8.15 The chin lift.

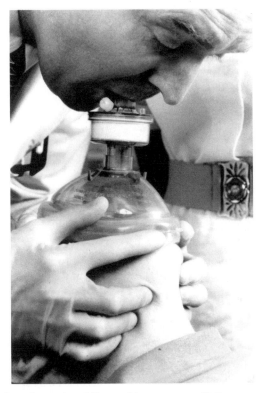

Figure 8.16 Use of a pocket mask to deliver positive-pressure ventilation.

sions are given for every one ventilation, with the person giving the cardiac massage counting aloud as he/she compresses the chest.

There are two key factors which determine a patient's chance of recovering from a cardiac arrest. First, the prompt initiation and efficiency of the basic life support provided by the dental surgeon and staff. Second, the speed at which expert help can be obtained. The survival of a patient following successful basic life support depends almost entirely on the speed at which the heart can be defibrillated. This is because the commonest type of cardiac arrest in adults is ventricular fibrillation. Early defibrillation (i.e. within minutes) provides the greatest chance of survival and thus it is essential to call for an ambulance as soon as a cardiac arrest is diagnosed.

Vasovagal syncope

The most frequent cause of collapse in the dental surgery is a vasovagal attack or faint. It can be initiated by anxiety, pain, hypotension, fatigue and occasionally fasting. Severely anxious and phobic patients undergoing sedation are especially prone to fainting. A vasovagal attack starts when a stimulus such as acute anxiety or pain produces a 'fight or flight' response. Due to vasodilatation, blood pools in the skeletal muscle and in the mesentery. In the absence of limb movements, venous return is reduced and consequently the cardiac output falls.

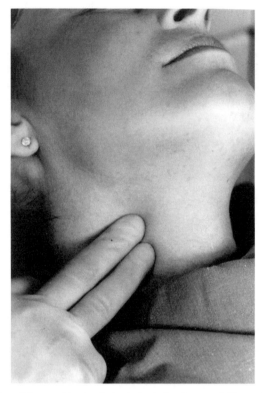

Figure 8.17 Palpation of the carotid pulse, just anterior to the sternomastoid muscle.

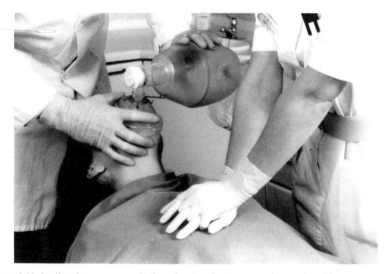

Figure 8.18 Cardiopulmonary resuscitation, showing chest compressions and positive-pressure ventilation.

Initially this may be offset by an increase in heart rate but if the venous return is still not restored, vagal decompensation occurs. This results in bradycardia, a reduction in cerebral blood flow and loss of consciousness.

The signs of an impending vasovagal attack include pallor, nausea, warmth, perspiration on the forehead and upper lip, and a rapid pulse. If the patient is not immediately treated they will rapidly lose consciousness and the pulse will become slow and weak. The pulse may fall as low as 30 beats per minute with significant periods of asystole. If treatment is delayed any further the patient may fit and become cyanotic.

Treatment involves laying the patient supine and raising the legs. Pregnant patients should be placed in the lateral position so that the weight of the foetus does not obstruct the inferior vena cava and thereby further reduce venous return. The airway should be maintained and oxygen administered via a face mask. The patient should recover rapidly. Once consciousness has been regained the patient should be reassured and a glucose drink given. If recovery is not rapid then the diagnosis should be reconsidered, whilst the airway and oxygenation are maintained. There is some evidence that atropine (0.6 mg) is useful in treating severe and prolonged faints but it should not be used routinely.

Vasovagal syncope can largely be prevented by laying the patient supine before commencing treatment and particularly prior to venepuncture. If this is not possible then the patient must be observed closely for the premonitionary signs of a vasovagal attack. If any occur the patient must immediately be laid supine. Sometimes it is possible to mistake vasovagal syncope from the effects of over-sedation. If a patient suddenly loses consciousness during the induction or maintenance of sedation, there should be a high index of suspicion that a vasovagal attack has occurred and appropriate treatment should be instituted.

Hypoglycaemia

Hypoglycaemia is the commonest cause of diabetic coma and can occur in patients with diabetes mellitus. It can be initiated by a missed meal, excessive anxiety or the presence of infection. All patients with diabetes mellitus undergoing dental care should be treated with caution and the dental surgeon should always be alert to the possibility of hypoglycaemia. The initial signs of hypoglycaemia are irritability, aggression and lack of co-operation. The patient will have cold, clammy skin and will start to become drowsy and disorientated. This will be followed by a gradual loss of consciousness despite a rapid and often full pulse. Whilst patients remain conscious, they should be given glucose or dextrose drink, tablets or gel by mouth. If they become unconscious intramuscular glucagon (1 mg/1 ml) or intravenous glucose (50 ml of a 50% solution) should be administered. The airway must be maintained and oxygen administered. Recovery should be rapid, whereupon consideration should be given to having the patient transferred to hospital. If a diabetic patient undergoing sedation becomes unconscious, glucose should be administered immediately via the intravenous cannula. If hypoglycaemia was the cause of unconsciousness recovery will be rapid. If the patient was hyperglycaemic (which is an unlikely cause of unconsciousness) and the diagnosis wrongly made, the consequences of giving glucose would not be severe although they may subsequently require insulin to reverse them. The converse situation of administering insulin to a patient who is hypoglycaemic is likely to be fatal!

Anaphylaxis

Anaphylactic shock is a massive allergic reaction caused by exposure to an antigen in a previously sensitised individual; occasionally the recipient is unaware of his/her sensitivity. True anaphylaxis is not mediated through histamine release although raised histamine levels are a feature of anaphylaxis. In dentistry, the most likely cause is an allergy to an antibiotic, especially penicillin or its derivatives, although milder skin-type allergies are more common. However, anaphylactic reactions can be initiated by a range of antigenic stimuli, including local anaesthetic solutions, intravenous drugs and even rubber gloves. A history of known allergies should be taken from the patient prior to commencing treatment.

The signs of an acute anaphylactic reaction are acute breathing difficulties, with bronchospasm and wheezing, flushing and oedema of the face and neck, and paraesthesia around the mouth and fingers. There will be severe hypotension and a rapid but weak or sometimes impalpable pulse, pallor, cyanosis and loss of consciousness. Treatment of anaphylaxis must be immediate. The patient should be laid flat with the legs raised. Adrenaline (1 mg/1 ml, 1 in 1000) should be administered intramuscularly or subcutaneously. The airway should be maintained and oxygen administered. If bronchospasm persists a further injection of adrenaline should be given. Expert emergency assistance should be summoned and hydrocortisone sodium succinate (200 mg) and chlorpheniramine maleate (10–20 mg) should be administered intravenously or intramuscularly. The possibility that cardiac arrest may supervene must always be considered.

Adrenal shock

Patients with adrenal disease or who are on long-term steroid therapy can suffer from adrenal shock in a stressful situation. Those presenting for sedation are at particular risk because of the high level of inherent anxiety or fear. The signs of adrenal shock are pallor, a rapid weak pulse, hypotension and ultimately loss of consciousness. Treatment should commence by laying the patient flat with the head down. The airway should be maintained and oxygen delivered via a face mask. Hydrocortisone sodium succinate (200 mg) should be administered intravenously or intramuscularly. If there is no improvement further doses of hydrocortisone should be administered until 500 mg has been given, when the diagnosis should be reconsidered. An emergency ambulance should be summoned.

A patient who is potentially at risk from adrenal shock should be given steroid cover prior to treatment under sedation. This will minimize the likelihood of an adrenal crisis occurring during treatment. If the patient does become unconscious during sedation then further hydrocortisone should be administered immediately. Patients who receive steroid therapy are at greater risk of steroid crisis and this should always be considered when a medical history is taken. The use of potent skin preparations or even steroid inhalers is frequently omitted from consideration and the potential risk of these products needs to be highlighted.

Epilepsy

Two forms of epilepsy are generally recognized—petit mal and grand mal. The former usually results in little more than a transient loss of consciousness for a relatively short period. True epileptic fits usually occur in known epileptics who have a poorly-controlled drug regimen. Fits may be precipitated by stress, anxiety and starvation and are thus more likely in patients who are undergoing sedation. The signs of an epileptic fit are loss of consciousness and rigid extended limbs, followed by jerking movements and sometimes incontinence or cyanosis. The fits are followed by a slow recovery and confusion. Treatment is aimed at protecting patients from injury and placing them in the recovery position. The airway should be maintained and oxygen administered.

If status epilepticus occurs, with persistent fitting lasting over 5 minutes or with signs of significant respiratory compromise, diazepam emulsion (10 mg) should be administered by slow intravenous injection. Theoretically the incidence of fits occurring during benzodiazepine sedation should be low because of the anticonvulsant effect of the benzodiazepines. However, there have been a number of reports of fits arising during midazolam sedation, mainly in poorly controlled epileptics. Caution should therefore be exercised when considering sedation for patients with a history of epilepsy. Fits can also occur in patients who lose consciousness for any other reason, especially those who faint and who are not immediately placed in a supine position.

Acute chest pain

Acute chest pain is usually caused by angina but the possibility of a myocardial infarction should always be considered. Angina results from myocardial ischaemia caused by narrowing of the coronary arteries. The demands of the heart increase during exercise, stress or hypertension and it is these situations which are most likely to precipitate an angina attack. Patients with dental anxiety undergoing sedation are more at risk. The features of an angina attack are a severe retrosternal pain radiating down the left arm and an irregular pulse. Sublingual glyceryl trinitrate, either in the form of tablets (0.5 mg) or spray (0.4 mg), should be administered and the airway should be maintained and oxygen given. If there is no relief in 3 minutes, the possibility of a myocardial infarction should be considered.

A myocardial infarct is caused by complete occlusion of a coronary artery, leading to sudden ischaemia and irreversible damage to part of the heart muscle. The patient will have severe crushing, retrosternal chest pain. He/she will be pale and cyanosed, breathless and may vomit. The pulse will be weak and irregular. The patient should be allowed to find the most comfortable position to minimize the pain and this will usually be in the seated position. Patients should not be reclined unless they lose consciousness since this increases the venous return and hence the cardiac output thereby making more demands on the oxygen-starved myocardium. Nitrous oxide 50% with oxygen 50% (if available) should be administered to relieve pain and anxiety. Aspirin (300 mg) should be given orally and the emergency services should be summoned. The patient must be closely monitored for any deterioration, particularly cardiac arrest, in which case cardiopulmonary resuscitation should be initiated.

Asthma

Asthma is a very common condition which varies considerably in severity. An acute asthma attack may be precipitated by anxiety, infection, exercise or sensitivity to allergen or irritant. The commonest signs of an asthma attack are breathlessness, with wheezing on expiration. Another presentation of asthma is of severe uncontrollable coughing with progressive difficulty in breathing. In either case the mainstay of treatment is to reassure the patient and allow them to maintain a position most comfortable for breathing. Oxygen and a salbutamol inhaler or nebulizer should be administered. If there is no improvement or if the attack turns into *status asthmaticus* the emergency services should be called. Oxygenation should be maintained and hydrocortisone sodium succinate (200 mg) administered intravenously or intramuscularly. If consciousness is lost, subcutaneous adrenaline should be administered. In hospital, the treatment of severe asthma is the intravenous administration of adrenaline whilst directly observing the patient's ECG.

Cerebrovascular accident

A cerebrovascular accident (CVA) is a general term referring to any disorder which suddenly limits the brain's blood supply (including the membranes) usually as a result of ischaemia, rupture and haemorrhage or embolism. A stroke is a clinical term referring to a total or partial attack of weakness on one side of the body that frequently results from a CVA. It may be primary (when it can be caused by cerebral haemorrhage or thrombosis) or secondary (when the primary disease is in the heart or blood vessels and an embolism or severe ischaemia occur secondarily). The patient will often complain of a sudden headache and may have dysarthria (unclear speech) or aphasia (inability to speak). There will be some degree of hemiplegia (partial or complete paralysis of one side of the face and/or body) and there may be loss of consciousness. The patient should be laid flat with the head down. The airway should be maintained and oxygen administered. Respiration must be monitored and assisted ventilation commenced if breathing ceases. The emergency services should be summoned.

Local anaesthetic toxicity

Toxic reactions from local anaesthetics can be caused by intravascular injection, excessively rapid injection or drug overdose. Patients may complain of light-headedness and visual or hearing disturbances. They may become agitated, confused and have difficulties in breathing. Severe toxicity reactions can cause convulsions, coma, respiratory arrest and cardiovascular collapse. The initial management should be to stop the local anaesthetic injection, maintain the airway and give oxygen. If the patient has a convulsion which does not resolve when in the supine position, diazepam emulsion (10 mg) should be administered by slow intravenous injection. The emergency services must be summoned and the patient monitored continuously for cardiac arrest.

Although sedation itself actually reduces the probability of an acute exacerbation of many specific medical conditions, patients undergoing sedation, because of their acute anxiety, are particularly at risk from stress-related medical emergencies. The dental surgeon who provides sedation must be constantly alert to the possibility of an emergency occurring before, during or after sedation. Distinguishing medical emergencies from sedation-related emergencies is essential, as is the competent management of both. Regular training and practice in procedures for the management of emergencies and in basic life support is essential for the whole dental team.

Local complications

A number of local complications can occur with intravenous sedation. The most common problem is extravenous injection. This happens when the cannula either fails to penetrate the lumen of the vein or completely transects the vein. In both cases the cannula will become located in the subcutaneous tissues. Flushing with 0.9% saline will clearly indicate if the cannula is not in the lumen of the vein. Saline will pool subcutaneously and a clear lump will be visible (Figure 8.19). If this occurs the cannula should be removed and re-sited elsewhere. If there is no sign of extravasation the sedation agent can be administered. Should any sedation agent be accidentally deposited in the subcutaneous tissues, the injection should be stopped and the area massaged to disperse the drug. Small quantities of extravenous midazolam usually disperse freely and cause no residual problems. An acute inflammatory reaction may occur with extravenous injection of diazepam but it is not usually necessary to administer vasodilators. Rarely, if an excessive amount of fluid is forced into the subcutaneous tissues, skin necrosis results (Figure 8.20).

Intra-arterial injection is a rare complication of intravenous sedation. Accidental cannulation of an artery should be avoided by good venepuncture technique. Veins should be selected well away from vital structures. The dorsum of the hand is the first choice for venepuncture because all the arteries of that region lie on the ventral surface. If it is necessary to use the antecubital fossa, only superficial veins lateral to the biceps tendon should be used, thereby avoiding the brachial artery and median nerve. All veins should be palpated prior to venepuncture to check for lack of pulsation. At venepuncture the colour

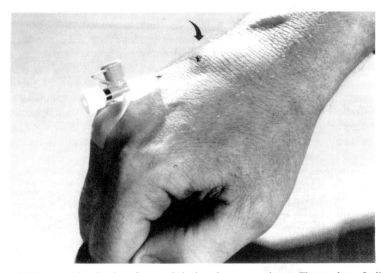

Figure 8.19 Incorrect localization of a cannula in the subcutaneous tissues. The test dose of saline has produced a lump which indicates pooling in the subcutaneous tissues.

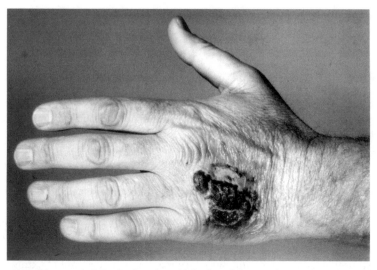

Figure 8.20 Skin necrosis following intradermal injection of diazepam in propylene glycol. This should have been avoided by careful observation of the injection site and discontinuation of the injection when the patient complained of pain.

of the flashback should be observed, bright red blood indicating that an artery has been penetrated. Intra-arterial cannulation is painful and injection of a test dose of saline will produce discomfort radiating down the arm. At the first sign that an artery may have been entered the injection must be terminated immediately. Pressure should be applied to the site and the arm elevated to prevent the formation of a large haematoma.

The main problem with intra-arterial injection is the potential for subsequent arterial spasm caused by the administration of irritant sedative drugs. Brachial artery spasm is a dangerous condition characterized by an intense burning pain radiating down the arm. The skin blanches and the radial and ulnar pulses weaken to the point of absence. Unless quickly treated the static blood coagulates, causing thrombosis, ischaemia and ultimately gangrene. Treatment relies on leaving the cannula in place and administering procaine (1%) in order to promote vasodilatation and to provide local analgesia. The patient should be immediately transferred to hospital where various surgical techniques, the administration of intravenous heparin or sympathetic blockade may be attempted if the spasm has not resolved. Thankfully the most widely used current sedation agent, midazolam, causes minimal vessel irritation and is unlikely to cause any significant problem if injected into an artery.

Good venepuncture technique is essential to avoid postoperative haematoma and thrombophlebitis. Many patients develop a haematoma at the site of cannulation (Figure 8.21). This can be prevented by careful venepuncture technique and ensuring that firm pressure is applied to the puncture wound after removal of the cannula. Poor technique, a damaged cannula, excessively rapid injection or use of an irritant sedation agent can cause significant vein damage and predispose to thrombophlebitis. The signs of thrombophlebitis can occur from days to weeks after the sedation appointment. Patients normally present with oedema, inflammation and pain over the course of the vein which was used for

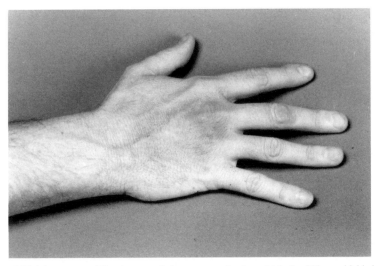

Figure 8.21 A haematoma following cannulation—a complication which should be avoidable in the vast majority of patients.

cannulation. The infected vein may feel hard and raised. Thrombophlebitis usually improves spontaneously over several weeks. The patient should be kept under review and reassured accordingly until the infection has completely resolved.

Finally, sedation patients must be appropriately protected from injury during sedation and recovery. Although sedated patients are conscious, they are less likely to take avoiding action if presented with a noxious stimulus. Protective glasses must be worn by the patient during operative dentistry to prevent dental instruments or materials causing an eye injury. The patient's limbs must be adequately protected from damage caused by equipment such as the bracket table. All electrical equipment must be earthed and no water spray must come into contract with any source of electricity otherwise there is a risk of electrocution. A naked flame must not be used where oxygen is present as this can cause an explosion. When patients are moved into the recovery area they must be watched and supported to prevent them from injuring themselves by falling over or hitting sharp objects. It is the responsibility of the dental surgeon to ensure that the sedated patient is protected from accidental injury. Careful instruction must also be given to the escort, who will assume responsibility for the patient from the time of leaving the surgery until full recovery from the effects of the sedation.

References and further reading

Edmondson, H.D. (1989). Medical emergencies in dental practice: an update on drugs and the management of acute airway obstruction. *Dental Update*, **16**, 254–255.

Edmondson, H.D. and Frame, J.W. (1986). Medical emergencies in general practice. 1. Acute medical problems, 2. Cardiopulmonary emergencies. *Dental Update*, **13**, 211–220, 263–273.

Resuscitation Council UK (1997). Guidelines for basic and advanced life support. UK Resuscitation
    Council, London.
Evans, T.R. (1990). *ABC of Resuscitation*. London: British Medical Journal.
Malemud, S.F. (1993). *Medical Emergencies in the Dental Office*. St Louis: Mosby.

9

Medicolegal and ethical considerations

Introduction

This chapter introduces some of the medicolegal and ethical issues that surround sedation and the practice of dentistry related to it. It is impossible to try and cover the subject anything other than superficially and there are several medicolegal textbooks which deal more with the specifically legal matters. It does not require too much skill, however, to observe that medicolegal issues are a growing and often unwelcome intrusion into modern clinical practice. In general terms, it is also true to say that the more a profession is regulated and subject to statute, the more it is liable to litigation. It is, therefore, important to understand the processes of law and the way in which they operate.

There are two parallel legal systems in Britain—the criminal system and the civil system. In the former, charges are usually heard in the magistrates and crown courts and the issue at stake is on the question of guilt. The choice of court is usually dependent on the seriousness of the charge and prosecutions may start in a lower court before being transferred to a higher court. In the civil system, small claims are usually heard in the county courts whilst the High Courts oversee all the lower courts. In civil cases the question concerned is of injury to the person or his property and the issue to be determined is whether or not compensation should be paid. Cases will be heard by a judge or registrar (a junior judge) and there will be no jury present. Dentists, therefore, face the possibility of actions in either the criminal or the civil systems. There are fundamental differences between the courts and the ways they work and there are differences within the United Kingdom, particularly in Scotland which has its own judicial system. As implied earlier, one of the principal differences is on the question of guilt. In the Criminal Courts, the concept of guilt is absolute; a person is either guilty or not guilty and will be judged and punished accordingly. Mitigating factors may be taken into account but in general terms these relate to the circumstances surrounding a situation rather than the details of the crime itself.

In the civil courts the issue of the balance of probability is taken into account and compensation determined accordingly. There are appeal systems for both the criminal and civil courts both referred to as the Court of Appeal although it is actually composed of two distinct courts. In neither case are witnesses called but rather legal arguments are put forward as to why the original decision was wrong. Finally, appeals against the decisions of the Court of Appeal can be made to the House of Lords although this has to be applied for (or 'leave given') and these are usually only allowed on contentious issues. Clinical staff are therefore well advised to understand the basic principles of law and how they may be affected by any charges brought against them. In this regard, both patient and dentist have certain rights and responsibilities and these are considered below. The European Court of Justice also has a duty to oversee the legal structures of member countries to ensure that the law is being applied fairly in member states. In other countries, legal systems vary considerably and the differing ways of administering the law can have a profound effect on the way justice is determined.

Rights and responsibilities of a patient

The primary and fundamental rights of all patients relate first to the principle of self determination (autonomy) and secondly to the expectation that any medical or surgical intervention offered should, above all else, safeguard the health of the recipient. In general terms this means that the benefit of any procedure should substantially outweigh any associated risks. In extreme cases, for example where a potentially life-saving operation may carry a high risk of mortality, the patient should be aware of the consequences of either intervening or not intervening. In essence this is the basis on which the principle of consent operates and this is explained more fully below. It does require of all health professionals that they always put the patients' interest first and that they do not let themselves become unduly influenced by their own personal preferences. A classic example where this approach can be seen to be lacking at times, is in oncology clinics where the views of radiotherapists and surgeons on the treatment of cancer frequently appear divergent and are not always related to best-known clinical practice. Similarly with the requirements for sedation, the patient's best interests must be served by any decision to recommend or withhold the offer of sedation. In this regard the concept of the 'sedation practice', where everybody has sedation all the time, is not a good one. It is self-evident that any patient who does not require sedation for a particular procedure should not have it offered or administered.

Patients also have the right to expect expert advice. Because of the privileged nature of the dental profession and its protected status in law, patients must be given appropriate, accurate and current information regarding any condition they have or treatment they are to receive. This can only be achieved by practitioners keeping up-to-date with modern developments through education and self improvement. Where a dentist is unable to provide accurate details on a relevant subject the information should be obtained from a third party.

This combination of expert advice based on safeguarding the patient's health as a primary responsibility should automatically lead to the third area of expectation, i.e. the receipt of quality care. Quality care is difficult to define but readily understandable. It is the prospect of having treatment which will be both effective and durable. There can be little doubt that the majority of all dental treatment performed in this country fits the above criteria but there are times when this is not the case. On occasion this may be due to inadequate treatment or failed materials and sometimes it is due to mistakes being made.

Surprisingly the law does not deny the likelihood of mistakes occurring but it does expect mistakes to be corrected and patients can anticipate the support of the law in this regard. The question as to whether a 'mistake' is of such severity that it would be considered negligent is not the same issue. The primary question in law to be answered first is whether the practitioner making the mistake was using reasonable skill when the accident occurred and second, was the opportunity given to remedy the error. Many cases have been lost by plaintiffs on this latter point. Plaintiffs in negligence cases also have a duty to submit themselves for examination by an expert witness for the defence if required so to do. This is supposed to prevent the malicious pursuit of a claim against a practitioner when, if such access were not agreed, the patient could effectively frustrate a reasonable defence. The same principle would apply to any medical records held on behalf a patient which may relate to an incident and these can be requested by the defendant or the plaintiff.

Duties and responsibilities of the dentist

The converse of the above section clearly applies. In delivering care to patients the dentist must safeguard their health, provide them with expert information, deliver quality care and remedy any mistakes which may occur. What a dentist does **not** have to do, is to conform to a single opinion with reference to a particular technique, method or procedure. There may even be disagreements on the matter of diagnosis and again this possibility is recognized by the courts. The law provides specific protection in this regard and the test applied is known as the *Bolam Principle*. This is that one cannot be guilty of negligence providing that the action taken is one which is in accordance with a practice accepted as proper by a responsible body of (medical/dental) opinion, even though another body of opinion may take a contrary view. With reference to the degree of skill required by the practitioner the test is the 'standard of the ordinary skilled man exercising and professing to have that particular skill'. In simple terms this eliminates the need for everyone to be 'best'. There is a need to be 'good enough' and what constitutes 'good enough' is effectively defined by the body of opinion of the particular specialty. (In Ireland the situation is slightly complicated because the plaintiff could still prove liability on the part of the dentist if it could be shown that despite a practice being accepted it had obvious and inherent defects and a recent case in Britain has adopted a similar view.) It would be true to say, however, that the majority of medicolegal problems today are associated with issues relating to negligence and the question of consent.

The dentist has an absolute duty to obtain the consent of a patient prior to undertaking any procedure. Failure to do so may constitute both assault and battery although, in reality, charges of this nature are usually rejected by the courts in favour of negligence claims. The whole question of consent is extensive and is dealt with in a later section of this chapter.

In addition to the legal constraints outlined above, the dentist also has other duties that would reasonably be expected of him/her. These include, for example the keeping of good, accurate and contemporaneous records. This is a common area of inadequacy and one which is frequently compounded by the retrospective addition of notes when problems occur. These are normally added in an attempt to clarify details but they have little standing in law and can make the defence of a case untenable. Notes must, therefore, be made as contemporaneously as possible but never to the detriment of clinical practice.

The notes made by a dentist and all the other information gathered about patients is confidential and there are very few occasions when it can be legally disclosed without the patient's consent. The right of confidentiality is well understood in law and can only be breached in well-defined circumstances. Dental records must therefore be kept promptly, accurately and confidentially.

The final area of responsibility of a dentist is that of observing legal and professional restraints. The law may influence clinical practice in a variety of ways, some obvious and some remote. It may seem strange for instance that a person should have his/her name removed from the dental register for an alcohol-related driving offence whereas one would probably anticipate the worst for sexually assaulting a patient. The law exists to protect the patient and its influence is profound, perhaps no more so than in the Dental Act which gives statutory powers to the General Dental Council (GDC). In other countries other regulatory bodies exist with varying degrees of power. In the UK, however, the GDC issues professional guidance and, with regard to sedation, its recommendations are quite specific. The dentist has a duty to observe the guidance given by the Council and failure to do so may result in a charge of professional misconduct and the dentist will have to provide answer to any such charges. On a more positive note, however, the GDC provides professional recognition for the dentist and it has enormous powers to stop the misappropriate use of dentistry.

Further restraints and guidance can be imposed by all sorts of 'unexpected' bodies including the fire services, the Health and Safety Executive, etc. and the modern dentist is faced with a plethora of often unwelcome intrusion into his/her clinical practice. None the less, it behoves everybody to be aware of the prevailing conditions and to pay due attention to their requirements.

Criminal and civil charges

The terms 'assault' and 'battery' are frequently used and poorly understood! Assault is technically the threat of violence against a person rather than the act of violence itself. Battery may be defined as any unwarranted physical contact but usually refers to an act that violates somebody. A person cannot be guilty of battery if he/she can prove that the contact was entirely accidental or that he/she was acting with the person's agreement. In some medicolegal cases some plaintiffs have tried to bring criminal proceedings claiming assault and battery based on technical questions of consent but this has rarely been successful. The Courts have usually decreed that claims for medical accidents should be heard under charges of negligence, i.e. as a civil claim rather than a criminal offence. This may have some advantages but for the patient, it does mean that until they go to court and successfully prove that negligence has occurred, it is impossible to know whether they are entitled to any compensation. In order to successfully prove negligence, a plaintiff must show:

a) that a duty of care was owed;
b) that the duty of care was breached;
c) that the breach in care resulted in harm to the patient.

Patients usually have no problem in proving the duty of care was owed (point a) but to prove points b and c simultaneously is not always easy. This sometimes leads to decisions which, to say the least, seem arbitrary.

In some cases the question of negligence is highly controversial and the court system is both expensive and unpredictable. Because of this there has been a considerable amount of criticism of the litigation system and in some countries 'no-fault' compensation schemes exist for medical accidents where compensation is awarded on fixed scales of payments but where the plaintiff does not have to prove negligence after a medical accident in order to get compensation. It could be argued that such a scheme is preferable although there are also opponents to such systems who argue that it could lower professional standards.

Consent

'Consent' is a noun to which various adjectives have been added including valid, informed, legal, implied, written, expressed, verbal, etc. The use of the adjectives, whilst commendable in attempting to clarify the position, frequently has the opposite effect and obscures the fundamental situation underlying the principle of consent. This is based on an ethical issue that would give competent patients (see below) the rights of self-determination. A person may choose without undue pressure to give or withhold consent to any examination, investigation or treatment as a matter of choice. If a patient has given his or her consent to a procedure being undertaken there can be no grounds for bringing a charge of battery (although they may still be able to claim the tort of negligence). In a court of law, therefore, the issue is simply one of whether a patient had consented and the practitioner has to be able to demonstrate that this was the case.

In some cases this may be possible simply by referring to the actions of the patient, for example, lying in a dental chair and opening one's mouth is almost certainly sufficient evidence of a patient consenting to an oral examination. No written signature is necessary in such cases but conversely, a signature obtained on an illegible consent form is unlikely to be acceptable evidence of consent in a complex restoration case carried out under intravenous sedation. This is because the dentist has a duty of care to the patient to explain, in such a way that the patient understands, the nature of the procedure being proposed, its associated risks and benefits **and** any possible alternative treatments. Modern consent forms nearly always include a section which is signed by practitioners certifying that they have explained the details to the patient. A move towards witnessed forms is also becoming more apparent and this may well become commonplace in the future. Even so, it should be remembered that the consent form in itself is not necessarily sufficient evidence of consent being obtained.

There is also the question of how much information should be given and this is not defined in law. Two classic cases are often quoted in the legal literature with reference to this: the *Sidaway* case and the *Bolam* case. Returning to the latter case again, Mr Bolam was given electroconvulsive therapy (ECT) to treat depression. As a result he sustained two fractures and sued his doctor for negligence especially as the doctor was aware of the risk and failed to warn him. The judge found in favour of the defendant, arguing that the doctor had complied with accepted medical opinion and that for Mr Bolam to succeed in his action he would have also have to have shown that he would not have proceeded with treatment had he been made aware of the risks of treatment. In

Mrs Sidaway's case, she was tragically paralysed by surgery to her back but again judgement went against her claim against the surgeon because the degree of risk was low and a body of neurosurgeons would not have routinely warned patients of the possibility of paralysis.

In defining how much information a patient should be given, therefore, this judgement sets out the principle, i.e. enough for the patient to make an informed decision. It is, therefore, probably not necessary to warn every patient that they have a one in half a million (or whatever, there being no accurate estimate available at the present time) chance of dying from sedation but it is probably negligent to fail to warn a patient of a possible numb lip after surgically removing a deeply impacted second premolar. The question of a person's age is also relevant to the laws of consent. The law defines adulthood from the date of a person's eighteenth birthday. From that age, providing they have the capacity to make decisions on their own behalf, people are said to be competent. In order to be deemed competent, an adult must be able to understand the proposed treatment in relation to its benefits and risks, to understand the alternative treatments available and the consequences of not accepting the proposals should they so choose. They must then be able to retain the relevant information long enough to make a free decision, i.e. with no external pressure from any interested party.

The law is complicated for children between the ages of 16 and 18 years and even more so for those under 16 years. In essence, however, the same general principles hold true for children when they consent (agree) to treatment. In the past, it has been traditional to ask parents to sign consent on behalf of their children under the age of 16 but, in law, children may now legally sign consent for both surgery and sedation if they are competent to do so. The age at which they become competent is not defined but it can no longer be set rigidly at age 16 and children below that age may legally consent to treatment. When there is conflict between the wishes of a parent and a child, the legal concerns will always centre around the best interests of the children and whether they were able to make a fully informed and understood decision.

If children refuse to consent to treatment, however, their parents may well have a legal right to overrule their refusal. This is unquestionably so with young children but must be exercised with progressive caution as children get older. The same rights can be given to the Courts in making a child a Ward of Court but such actions need to be taken with some sensitivity and are normally only appropriate in life-threatening situations. Consent may also be given by legal guardians, adoptive parents and the local authorities for children who are the subject of a care order.

In all cases where sedation is being administered, consent should be given freely and recorded on a standard form (Figure 9.1). In cases where issues may arise (e.g. the refusal to consider blood transfusions), a modified form can be used which specifically details any limitation of consent.

Finally, the hardest area in the question of consent is probably in relation to those adult patients who are not deemed competent. At the current time nobody can authorize consent on behalf of an incompetent adult and doctors and dentists must act in their patient's best interests, wherever possible obtaining two independent professional views as to the advisability of any proposed treatment. The practitioner's overriding responsibility is the duty of care which is owed to the patient and, if necessary, this should be demonstrable to a court of law.

CONSENT FOR TREATMENT UNDER SEDATION

NAME   ....

ADDRESS ....

....

D. o. B.   ....

PROCEDURE:

PATIENT
    (Only sign this section if the information is correct
        and you understand it.)
I am the patient/parent/guardian** and agree to the treatment
proposed and explained to me by.................. . I agree to the
use of sedation and local anaesthetic. I understand that the
procedure may not be carried out by the dentist who has been
treating me so far. I confirm that I have been given the
opportunity to ask questions.

Signed.......................   Date...............

DENTIST
I confirm that I have explained the procedure and the
anaesthetic/sedation in a way which I believe is understood.

Signed.......................   Date ....

**Delete as necessary

Figure 9.1 A standard consent form. Modified forms can be used for patients who wish to withhold consent for some aspects of their treatment.

Parents may give consent on behalf of children between the ages of 16 and 18 years when the child is not deemed competent to do so.

In the UK there are also some exceptions to the laws regarding consent for patients who are subject to certain orders under the Mental Health Act of 1983. However, these and other such details are well explained in various medicolegal textbooks and in the MDU/DDU booklet on the subject of consent.

Risk assessment

Risk assessment is essentially a management tool, used to minimize the incidence of untoward events but it can be applied to clinical situations with great effect. It is closely linked with issues of quality and the ever-increasing need to demonstrate that standards are high and improving. It is a process which should be proactive and not reactive, i.e. it should attempt to stop mistakes before they happen rather than using the mistakes themselves as the drivers of change.

Figure 9.2 illustrates the sort of areas that can be considered in risk assessment. They should be dealt with systematically and repeated periodically. Any problems identified should be addressed and solutions put in place which should themselves be assessed after a period of time. For risk assessment to operate satisfactorily, members of staff must 'own' the process and feel that it is in all their interests to strive for continued improvement. If this is achieved, hopefully the last section of this book will be irrelevant.

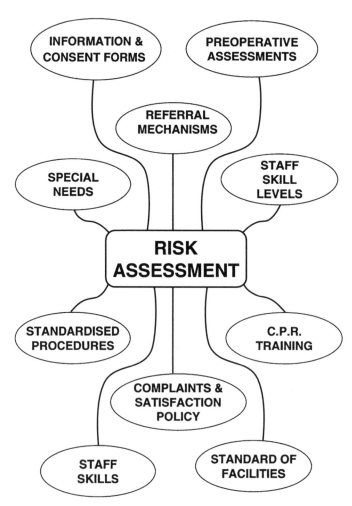

Figure 9.2 Some of the factors to be considered as part of a risk assessment. The list is not exclusive and needs to be adapted to the particular circumstances of each situation.

And if the worst happens?

The incidence of complications from patients undergoing simple sedation for dental treatment is extremely low. However, there have been several critical episodes some of which have unfortunately been fatal. In such cases there will be a sequence of procedures to be followed and questions to be asked. The purpose of this is to establish:

1. What went wrong and why did it go wrong?
2. Had a proper pre-assessment procedure been followed?
3. Was the sedation technique used justifiable and correctly administered by a competent person?
4. Were the appropriate support staff available at all times?
5. Was a correct resuscitation procedure followed by staff who knew and performed their duties.
6. Were all the necessary drugs and equipment available?

If the dentist can give reason for the first question and answer the remaining questions positively, there will be little cause for concern. If not, the failings need to be identified so that the coroner can determine a verdict in relation to the patient's death and release the body for burial or cremation.

Fortunately most accidents are not fatal. It behoves everyone concerned with the practice of sedation to ensure that it is a safe, efficient and effective procedure which is undertaken for the benefit of the patient. In the vast majority of cases this will be beyond doubt; in the few cases where mishaps occur, careful and prompt management should ensure that a minor problem does not become a catastrophe—from either a clinical or a legal viewpoint! For most patients, conscious sedation enables them to undertake dental treatment which they would at best find uncomfortable and, at worst, impossible. For the dentist, it offers a set of tools which can aid in treatment provision and general patient management.

References and further reading

Bolam (1957). v. Friern Hospital Management Committee. 2 All ER 118. (1WLR582).

Dental Defence (1997). *Consent to Treatment*. London: Medical Defence Union.

Mental Health Act (1983). Code of Practice, see Chapter 15.

Sidaway (1985). v. Bethlem Royal Hospital Governors. 1 All ER 643 (2WLR480).

Appendix

Table of sedation-related drug generic and trade names and their function

Generic name	Trade name(s)*	Main function
Amethocaine	Ametop	Topical anaesthesia of the skin
Midazolam	Hypnovel	Sedation
Diazepam	Valium	Sedation
	Diazemuls	
Eutectic mixture of lignocaine/procaine	EMLA	Topical anaesthesia of the skin
Fentanyl (Alfentanil)	Sublimaze (Rapifen)	Opiate analgesia
Flumazenil	Anexate	Benzodiazepine antagonist
Naloxone	Narcan	Reversal of opiates
Promethazine	Medised, Phenergan, Phensedyl, Sominex	Oral sedation in children
Propofol	Diprivan	Anaesthesia, patient-controlled sedation
Temazepam	Temazepam	Oral sedation in adults
Triclofos	Triclofos	Oral sedation in children
Trimeprazine	Vallergan	Oral sedation in children

*Not all registered trade names are included for all drugs listed.

Index